Managing
Life with
Incontinence

Editors: Cheryle B. Gartley, Mary Radtke Klein,
Christine Norton, and Anita Saltmarche

D1257479

The Simon Foundation for Continence

Published by
The Simon Foundation
Post Office Box 815
Wilmette, IL 60091
www.simonfoundation.org

Project Credits
Project Manager: Jasmine Sassack
Book Designer: Maritza Medina
Illustrator: Nigel Webb

*The health information contained herein is provided for educational
and support purposes only and is not intended to replace discussions
with a health care provider. All decisions regarding your care must
be made with a health care provider, considering your unique
characteristics and health needs.*

ISBN-10: 0615602258
ISBN-13: 978-0-615-60225-7
Library of Congress Control Number: 2012934115
Printed in the United States of America

First Edition: March 2012

10 9 8 7 6 5 4 3 2 1

Thank You

This book was made possible by educational grants to
the Simon Foundation for Continence from:

Astellas USA Foundation

Hollister Incorporated

SCA Hygiene Products

Table of Contents

On the Nobility of Incontinence

Rick Rader, MD

When I grew up, guys' names had a ring about them. "Duke" still conjures up someone you want behind you in a schoolyard brawl, while "Spike" makes a decent back-up if Duke wimps out. You'd likely agree that "Rock" would be the one to call if you had to get your bike back from the kid who stole it; the delinquent thief's name would probably be something like "Biff" or "Mack." You definitely wouldn't feel confident with a "Stanley," "Bernie," or "Alfred" backing you up if you had to walk through a schoolyard claimed by a gang of guys wearing black leather jackets boasting their membership in the "Eastside Cut Throats" social club. Yeah, guys' names have a ring about them. But sometimes names don't pan out. Sometimes when you're looking for constructive help it doesn't come from the place you'd expect. "Alfred" is certainly not a power name like "Duke," "Spike," or "Rock." But a guy named Alfred became synonymous with power; he, in fact, unleashed power that the world had never known. In 1867 Alfred, a Swiss chemist, figured out that when nitroglycerin was mixed with an absorbent, inert substance it became stable and safer to handle. Realizing he was onto something marketable, he considered naming the powerful substance "Nobel's Safety Powder." Instead he settled on "dynamite," referring to the Greek word for power. And power was indeed what he amassed; power and fortune.

Thirty years later, Alfred Nobel signed his last will and testament, giving a large share of his fortune to fund a series of prizes bearing his name.

> The whole of my remaining realizable estate shall be dealt with in the following way: the capital shall be invested…, the interest on which shall be annually distributed in the form of prizes to those who, during the preceding year, shall have conferred *the greatest benefit on mankind…*; one part to the person who shall have made the most important discovery within the domain of *physiology or medicine…*

Thus the Nobel Prize in Medicine was first conferred in 1901. There is no doubt that this prize has served as a testimony to the greatest medical advances and researchers the world has seen. All game changers, without doubt: Koch's (1905) identification of the tubercle bacillus and related work on tuberculosis; Landsteiner (1930) on blood groups and blood typing; Fleming, Chain, and Florey (1945) for penicillin; Crick, Watson, and Wilkins (1962) on the discovery of DNA; Banting and Macleod (1923) for the discovery of insulin; Murray and Thomas (1990) on organ and cell transplantation. It is probable that anyone reading this page has benefited directly or indirectly from work related to one of the 102 Nobel Prizes awarded in medicine.

While the Nobel Prize in Medicine is certainly significant, why are we referring to it in an introduction to a book on incontinence? Answer: to make an important point. Help doesn't always come from the place you'd expect. A careful survey of the prizes reveals that not a single one has been given for any significant work in the treatment of incontinence. While each of us hopes a cure is still on some researcher's "bucket list," to date, there has not been any Prize-worthy "game changing" work on this condition. If we look to the big names right now, the Dukes, the Rocks, the Macks, and the Nobels, we find little concrete help.

But suppose, just suppose that there was a great advance. It's not so farfetched.

Recently Richard Craver, writing in the *Winston-Salem Journal*, reported that researchers at The Institute of Regenerative Medicine, Wake Forest University, produced the first functional anal sphincter in a laboratory setting. Ah the anal sphincter, both hero and culprit to us all.

When we're talking about a sphincter, we need to recognize we are at its mercy. Current treatments available for restoring damaged sphincters all have high complication rates and limited success. These sub-optimal treatments have included skeletal muscle grafts, injectable silicone material, or implantation of mechanical devices. No candidates here for a trip to Stockholm and a share of a $1.5 million Nobel Prize.

But now, according to Professor Khalil Bitar, one of the lead researchers involved in the work mentioned above, "In essence, we have built a replacement sphincter that we hope can one day benefit human patients. This is the first bioengineered sphincter made with both muscle and nerve cells, making it pre-wired for placement in the body."

If, in fact, a workable and sustainable bioengineered replacement sphincter could be perfected, how would it stack up for a Nobel Prize? It is hard to tell. Would it become a named advancement? Would capturing of the Nobel Prize make a difference in people's lives?

The fact is that we're not where we'd like to be with the science. We're not sure how soon we're going to get there. So, in the meantime, this book from the Simon Foundation engages the reader in the reality, the mythology, and the experience of living, fearing, cursing, adjusting to, and accepting the intrusion of a defiant sphincter and the prospect of adapting successfully to the "new new" that it imposes.

Incontinence and its impact are fairly complex, and I like simple. As a medical student "simple" was my ticket to appreciating the synergy of the body's complex systems. When we hit Chapter 26 of Guyton's physiology text (imagine no mention of "elimination" until chapter 26) I was confronted with some heavy-duty illustrations and intense physiological principles. I needed "simple."

I quickly realized that in the physiology of elimination the sphincter was the key. It was the body's equivalent to the ice hockey team's all-important goalie, with the puck representing both urine and feces. Take your eye off the puck and you're incontinent.

The "simple" (but eloquent) explanation for the role that the sphincter plays came to me by way of an unforgettable British physiology professor who stated:

> They say man has succeeded where the animal fails because of the clever use of his hands, yet when compared to the hands, the sphincter ani (anal sphincter) is far superior. If you place into your cupped hands a mixture of fluid, solid, and gas and then through an opening at the bottom you try to let only the gas escape, you will fail. But the anal sphincter can do it. The sphincter can apparently differentiate between solid, liquid, and gas. It apparently can tell whether its owner is alone or with someone, whether standing or sitting down, whether its owner has his pants on or off. No other muscle of the body is such a protector of the dignity of man, yet so ready to come to his relief.
>
> *As quoted from Dr. Walter C. Bornemeier*

Protector of the dignity of man for sure, but like Alfred's dynamite, the anal sphincter, and its urinary counterpart, also have the capacity to decimate and forever change the landscape. Too bad that adverse impact hasn't gotten more attention.

To answer the question as to whether a bio-engineered sphincter could walk away (maybe that's asking too much of any sphincter, natural or engineered) with the Nobel Prize and why the answer to that question is the rationale for this book, we have to look at popular culture and incontinence.

Incontinence remains one of the last stigmatized targets of a dysfunctional body system. The sociologist Erving Goffman described "stigma" as "spoiled identity." To be realistic, the working, functioning sphincter doesn't really have an identity. We don't characterize it; we see it neither as an unsung hero nor a team player. It simply exists without any persona. Perhaps its invisibility is a testimony to the hundreds of millions of lives in which it quietly goes about its business of "protecting the dignity of man." None of us sing praises to a hearty sphincter. If anything, we praise our own self-control (so little do we know about what is happening behind the scenes) in making it to the restroom in the nick of time. Muscles, hearts, erectile dysfunction, healthy lungs all get good face time. But in our culture, the sphincter has no advance men, no PR department, and no creative department ready to pitch an unforgettable tag line, no one to give it a pop personality.

But let it tire, fatigue, derail, or forget its ninja skills and it becomes not only apparent, but the center of attention. An impaired sphincter can reconfigure lives that were doing just fine before it abandoned its sentry post. It can redefine lives. Lives that never gave the darn "thing" (one does not want to personify a traitor) a thought, now must plan, scheme, schedule, prepare, anticipate, and compensate in ways that would impress Harry Potter.

In spite of the above, the unfortunate truth is that an announcement that a synthetic replaceable sphincter has been perfected would not raise an eyebrow at the Nobel Prize Nominating Committee. The simple fact is that in a world awash in information, there is no awareness, no notoriety, no celebrity spokesperson, no 10-K races, no walks, no symbolic ribbons, no sitcoms, no Hallmark cards, no bus posters, no highly visible centers of excellence, and no visibility for the impaired sphincter and its outcome, incontinence. Worse still is that there is no mandated curriculum in medical schools, never a question on board exams for doctors, no challenges to the interns on ward rounds, and very few support groups. There are more support groups for people who periodically misplace their car keys than for people with urinary or fecal incontinence. It is doubtful that any of this will change in the very near future. So, this book and the information that it both invites and provides is an attempt to fill the gap and hasten the change.

This book will help individuals with incontinence, their families, significant others, healthcare providers, policy makers, and perhaps songwriters, playwrights, and poets navigate the reconfigured lives that are possible for all of us.

As to my hope for the Nobel Prize Nominating Committee to one day recognize and celebrate either a cure or successful treatment for incontinence, I would like to refer back to the Prize medal itself and its irony. The medal of the Nobel Assembly at the Karolinska Institute depicts the Genius of Medicine holding an open book in her lap, collecting the water pouring out from a rock in order to quench the thirst of a sick girl at her side. If the image of water pouring onto a girl's lap is not reflective of incontinence I don't know what is. Maybe that's what we needed all along to spur the science in this area; for the Nobel Committee to read its own subliminal message, that cures must be found for incontinence.

Finally, in support of my argument for full Nobel recognition at the time a cure is announced, I present the inscription on the Nobel Prize medal, **"Inventas vitam juvat excoluisse per artes."** Loosely translated, "And they who bettered life on earth by their newly found mastery."

A fitting inscription for the person or persons who provide the definitive treatment for incontinence; until then, this book will be highly prized itself.

Is this Book for You?

If you, like millions worldwide, live with a misbehaving bladder and/or bowel (which healthcare professionals call intractable incontinence) you may react in a variety of ways to this symptom. For some, it is simply a matter of conducting a thorough search to find the optimal way to protect their clothing, furniture, and bedding. For others, the symptom of incontinence is life changing.

Research has shown that the psychological, emotional, and social impact of incontinence is often not correlated to the amount of leakage. You may leak just a small amount once a day and feel greatly distressed by this change in your body, while others may have substantial challenges with incontinence and yet find that few aspects of life are impacted by the leakage.

The authors of this book recognize that the symptom of incontinence affects each individual differently. However, it is our hope that by understanding the common reactions to a misbehaving bladder and/or bowel you will find within these covers solutions for living a life not hampered by restrictions. As you read through these chapters you may also recognize insidious ways in which your incontinence has limited your life without your realization.

This book is for those individuals who have sought professional medical attention for incontinence, but who are still living with the symptom of bladder or bowel leakage. So often we hear from people sentences that begin with "I used to": I used to sail, I used to go to church, I used to love to hike in the fall... If you find that "I used to" is a part of your vocabulary, then this book is for you.

How to Use This Book

This book was written by authors who know and understand that the impact of incontinence is powerful and can lead to many negative changes in your life—from discouragement, to living a life of self-imposed restrictions, to total isolation. We also know that improvement in your quality of life is possible if you are willing to do some work. You have to make the effort, but we believe that within these pages you will find some of the best tools to help you begin.

The two chapters on urinary and bowel incontinence provide some basic information on function, reasons for loss of control, and fundamental techniques for developing or maintaining the best control possible. The rest of the chapters look out to the broader world and not only provide information, but suggest strategies, techniques, and resources that you can put to work.

The editors recognize that not everything in this book will be of use to each reader. Some may find the book most helpful if they pick and choose what feels most applicable to their own life. To help you do this, we have written a preface before each chapter which will give you an overview of what is contained within. You may want to begin by reading each of these. Once you've read the editors' summaries you may decide to read the book in a completely different order than how it is set out—the sequence that best fits your needs and interests.

Because there are many experts who have contributed to this endeavor you may notice that the writing style changes from chapter to chapter. We have elected to let our readers enjoy these different voices. We also know that cultural differences will appear, especially when this book is translated into other languages; but we feel that the overarching commonality of reactions to and feelings about bladder and bowel problems transcends any differences there are between our cultures. Therefore we have not made any attempt to mitigate these differences through the editing process.

You may hear similar things from different authors. But each time you will be hearing it from a different perspective, and in a different context. If a concept or suggestion keeps recurring it is because we felt that our readers would find these different perspectives useful.

Between chapters you will find "Lived Experiences"—stories written by people from around the world who were willing to speak openly about their own experiences with incontinence. These personal glimpses are included not as models or ideals, but rather as a personalized look at the human experience and the universality of the struggle.

We are well aware that unknown numbers of individuals struggle with loss of both bowel and bladder control. However, the use of the phrase "bladder and/or bowel control" is awkward and therefore we hope that readers who are coping with both a misbehaving bladder and a misbehaving bowel will understand when they see a reference to either bladder or bowel control.

Please do not worry if when looking through this book for the first time you think this all looks like too much to tackle. You don't have to make changes overnight or commit to every technique or strategy. Take this in small bites. Build on and celebrate your successes and eventually, at your own pace, we hope bigger changes will come.

Some readers will just want to read and think about the content. Others will immediately want to work hard and do all the exercises included. Please feel free to copy these exercises for your personal use or to make notes in the book itself if it helps you to remember a good idea.

At the back of the book you will find a list of resources that includes organizations similar to the Simon Foundation for Continence from around the world; thus, via logging on to their websites you can find incontinence information in many different languages.

Most importantly, we hope that you enjoy this book. It is meant to help you see your incontinence in a different light, realize that you are not alone, that others have found some positive solutions, and encourage you to change the way you view yourself and how you want to live and contribute in the world.

CHAPTER 1

Understanding the Taboos About Bladders and Bowels

CHRISTINE NORTON, PhD, RN, LESLEY DIBLEY, MPhil, RN

EDITOR'S NOTE: This chapter discusses the possible reasons why bladder and bowel incontinence is so difficult to talk about and difficult to live with, and how this can lead to feelings of embarrassment and shame. If you are interested in this, you may also want to read Chapter 2 on the related topic of stigma. Drawing on evidence from psychology, sociology, and anthropology, we discuss the rules that societies have in relation to bladder and bowel control, and the effect these rules have on how we feel about our own control, or lack of it. Not everything that is discussed here will apply to all people in all circumstances, but we hope that if incontinence makes you feel bad, some of the ideas discussed here may help to give you some understanding of why you feel the way you do.

Humans are social beings, and children become socialised by learning the rules and boundaries set firstly by their parents or caregivers. As they grow, they merge into pre-school, education, and working life, learning the social rules and expectations along the way. These arbitrary rules are what bind societies and groups together, and everyone in that society or group recognises the rules as the expected way to do things. By learning and accepting the rules, the growing child becomes socialised into the world in which he or she grows up.

The point of these rules is that they provide some structure and order to the way we live; if most people did not follow the rules, there would be chaos. Some rules are based on moral and ethical principles – don't steal from others, don't be violent towards others – and become enforceable by law. Some moral and ethical rules are based on relationships – who can marry who, who can have sexual relationships with who, whilst other rules are in place to promote safety – drive on the correct side of the road, wear a safety belt, obey road signs, for example. Not all rules are there to control dangerous or law-breaking behaviours though. Some rules are better understood as manners, or appropriate ways of managing personal behaviour in public, and there are social rules about acceptable public eating, drinking, greeting each other, and toilet activities.

Because most of us obey most of the rules most of the time, society does not break down into disorder, and since we have all learnt these rules as children, they are so deeply ingrained that we do not have to think about them – we just know that some things are right and others are wrong. Rules are present in all societies and in some circumstances allow us to put out of our minds the more unpleasant issues within society that we tend not to want to think, much less talk, about. These issues, such as child sexual abuse, prostitution, or domestic violence may be seen as taboo.

The rules that govern our toilet behaviours are best described as manners and being continent is bound up in this deeply-ingrained knowledge of how to behave in society. The feelings of shame, guilt, embarrassment, and stigma, which can be associated with poor bladder and bowel control, arise from the inability to comply with these rules, even when you really want to be able to do so.

Manners

All societies have rules about how to manage personal behaviour in public, with very clear guidelines on what is and is not allowed. These often complex rules – or manners – are learnt by children and newcomers to the social group, and may include aspects such as how to eat and drink (using cutlery, elbows off the table) or how to greet each other (a handshake, a bow, a kiss on the cheek). It is often considered rude or discourteous not to comply with accepted manners. This often changes over time. For example, in Japan in the last century it was considered polite to cover the mouth with a hand to hide the sight of food entering the mouth or being chewed – this has now largely disappeared in public behaviour.

We may find that we have to temporarily adopt different manners when visiting another country in order to not cause offense to the society of which we have become a temporary member – bowing instead of shaking hands in some countries, and avoiding physical contact between men and women in others.

It seems that every society has rules about toilet behaviours, and in some social groups these may be related to hygiene as well as to manners. People who live in conditions with no formal sanitation and drainage, such as some remote villages in developing countries, have codes of behaviour about emptying the bladder or bowel. These activities are only allowed outside of living areas, usually well away from houses or villages, and often with separate areas for men and women.

Although bladder and bowel emptying is now considered a private activity in Western countries, this has not always been the case. Only a few hundred years ago it was acceptable behaviour in the street. Even the Romans, who built elaborate baths and sewers, had genuinely public toilets with no doors or privacy. The introduction of modern sanitation over the past 200 years, with flush toilets and main drains to carry the waste away unseen, has allowed most people to completely privatise their bladder and bowel function. It is usually done behind closed doors with nobody watching (or even hearing) what happens. Most adults have very little contact with the waste products of others, except that of their children during the first few years of the child's life. This private world means that most adults do not know what is "normal," and because we do not talk about it, few realise that many, many others also have problems.

In teaching toilet manners to our children we instil in them the social rules about polite toilet behaviour. We start toilet training by urging our children to let us know when they need to go to the toilet, but we gradually move them towards understanding that what they do in the toilet is private. We teach them the difference between appropriate and inappropriate toilet behaviour. Boys learn to stand to pass urine and sit to move the bowels. Girls learn to sit for both. We teach them to flush away the evidence afterwards because nobody else wants to see their waste. In achieving toilet training, children must learn to recognise and interpret the physical feelings associated with needing to pass urine or open the bowels, to understand how much time they have between the first physical feeling and needing to be in the bathroom, and how to control the need to empty the bladder or bowel until they are in an appropriate setting, as determined by the society in which they live. Above all, we teach children the importance of good control.

These ingrained behaviours are based on society's rules about toilet manners, and we expect to be able to comply; inability to do so causes distress for most people. We want to be able to use the toilet on our own and in private. It is one of the fears of becoming frail, unwell, or disabled – what if someone else needs to help me with getting onto the toilet, or to get clean afterwards?

Taboos

A taboo is a subject which is not talked about, usually because the truth is too unpleasant for people to acknowledge – such as incest. A taboo subject becomes an object of discomfort in a society that effectively ignores its presence by refusing to acknowledge or address it. Often this is because the society itself does not know how to respond.

Children learn about the notion of taboo when they learn that certain words and behaviours are considered rude, not nice, and not talked about. Many jokes amongst older children are focused on body function taboos, such as sexual activity and behaviour, as well as on bladder and bowel function.

Attitudes can change over time and subjects that were once taboo can become more acceptable. It is now easier to talk about sex and dying than it was fifty years ago. People are more aware of issues such as sexual abuse and sexually transmitted diseases, and previously unmentionable topics such as voluntary euthanasia (mercy killing) are receiving much more attention now. But bladders and bowels are still difficult to talk about. An article in UK *Vogue* fashion magazine (March 2010) was entitled "Poo – the last taboo," talking to women with bowel problems about why the subject is so difficult to address. This type of media coverage is rare, but helps raise awareness amongst the medically well population that poo causes problems for many otherwise healthy, successful, and active men and women.

We tend to try to avoid things which make us feel uncomfortable or that we interpret as being dirty or unpleasant. In relation to the human body, "dirty" may also mean moist and slimy, perhaps with an associated disagreeable odour. What makes something dirty depends also on the context. Dirt has often been called "matter out of place" and it is only when a substance is misplaced that it becomes offensive to the senses. Some body products are, in most societies, almost universally thought to be dirty – for example, feces, vomit, mucus, and saliva – as soon as they are outside of the body. Urine in your bladder or in the toilet bowl is fine. Urine on the floor, on a chair, or in the street is not. Saliva in your mouth is fine. Spitting in the street or dribbling is not. Similarly, most parents manage to change their babies' nappies without problems, but many people find that poo left smeared on a toilet seat or not flushed away is offensive to them. Body substances in some settings are not offensive – intimate contact with the body fluids of a lover causes us few problems, but contact with those same fluids from a stranger offends us.

> *Beauty is no quality in things themselves: It exists merely in the mind which contemplates them; and each mind perceives a different beauty.*
> —David Hume

Different societies and individuals have different interpretations of what is considered dirty, and respond to dirt in different ways. These social and individual interpretations are not always rational; although feces are contaminating, have an often unpleasant odour, and can potentially transmit disease, fresh urine smells very little and urine is sterile, so is therefore unlikely to pose any threat to health.

Shame and Guilt

Shame and guilt are complex emotions which arise in us when we know we have done something that we perceive to be wrong. Shame is "a painful mental feeling aroused by a sense of having done something wrong" whilst guilt is "a feeling that one is to blame for something." Both of these complex emotions arise internally when the person experiencing those feelings does something that they know, due to early childhood socialisation, is likely to be disapproved of. An individual's perceptions of what is right and wrong are deeply embedded in the rules by which they were raised – if anything happens to challenge those rules, the person feels bad, which results in the emotions of shame and guilt.

If we are unable to control our bladder or bowels, then we feel shameful and guilty because we have not been able to conform to the teaching of our early childhood, and we know, deep in our subconscious, that conformity equates with approval. Remember the praise and delight you gave to your children when they first performed on the potty, gaining control of bowel and then bladder? Childhood success in controlling bladder and bowel functions is positively reinforced by praise, reward, and encouragement from parents, and children learn to respond to this because, at that age, they want more than anything else in the world to please their parents. This early teaching and positive reward for conforming to social rules stays with us, even though we may not be able to consciously recall it or be aware of it.

Dealing With Shame and Guilt

Since shame and guilt arise when we cannot follow the social rules, a shift in under-standing is required to help you cope with these difficult feelings. You probably learnt your control in childhood (if you ever had it) when bladder and bowel were functioning normally. If these now do not function normally, you may be expecting too much of yourself to try and fulfill those early childhood social rules. By setting yourself some new social rules and managing your bladder and bowel in order to meet these rules, you can take charge of a new form of control and remove your feelings of shame and guilt. You can read about more ideas on how to manage these feelings in other chapters of this book.

Embarrassment

Embarrassment is a different matter altogether, because it depends on the expected or actual reactions of others for this emotion to arise. You do not usually feel embarrassed on your own – only when someone else reacts negatively (or might react negatively) to something you have done. We have all done something embarrassing – spilt coffee on the boss's desk, shown ourselves up in an important meeting, trailed toilet paper on our heels from the office washroom – but equally have learnt to cope with such episodes, otherwise we would all just stay at home.

To embarrass someone is to make them feel awkward or ashamed, and we experience embarrassment when others see or know (or might see or know) things about us that we would rather they did not know. We often feel embarrassed when we know that we have broken the rules learnt as children and when others witness this, because we have failed to project an acceptable self to others in a social situation. If you have a bowel accident at home you might feel shame or guilt, but you would only feel embarrassed if someone else in the house was aware of what had happened and they do, or might, express disapproval in some way.

We all recognise the symptoms of embarrassment – blushing, sweating, maybe a faster heart beat, feeling hot or cold, feeling flustered. This uncomfortable and unpleasant feeling arises from knowing you have transgressed a social rule, and that someone else may or will notice. For example, since we are all supposed to poo in private, many healthy "normal" adults have difficulty opening their bowels in public toilets, for fear of being overheard or making a smell. They fear that others in the washroom may react negatively, even if nothing is said, and they do not want to feel embarrassed. This kind of "body betrayal" gives us away by creating instances where others witness or know about the unspeakable yet normal functions of our bodies. Passing gas unintentionally, having others hear or smell urine or feces being passed, having a toilet that will not flush to remove body products are all commonly said to be embarrassing, depending on the situation. Even though everyone does these things, it is feared that if others know this about you, you will create a bad impression. Being obviously incontinent in public would make almost anyone feel embarrassed.

Some people feel most embarrassed not with strangers or close friends, but with acquaintances and individuals who are known, but not known very well. Strangers do not matter so much to many of us – we are likely to think that this person does not know us, is never likely to meet us again, and that it does not matter if they feel badly about us. Those closest to us who often know about the incontinence may no longer notice, and are certainly less likely to think badly about us if they do notice. We have the most risk of feeling embarrassed with those in our "mid-range" of relationships – those individuals with whom we would like to maintain our public face of control and respectability, such as work colleagues. We fear that such acquaintances will think less of us if we display unexpected traits such as poor bladder or bowel control.

We know that many people in the general population find the idea of others seeing, hearing, or smelling them passing urine or feces very embarrassing. All sorts of strange behaviours are developed to keep toilet use private and prevent others from witnessing these events, particularly in public restrooms and at work or at friends' houses. More women than men report feeling embarrassed in this way. This might be related to the actions each gender takes to pass urine or stool – men stand side by side at the urinal, and are socialised into passing urine in a setting which is less private than the single cubicle used by women who must sit down. Men can also easily pass urine discretely outside if necessary – behind a tree or shrub – whilst women do not have this option. These factors may explain, in part, the different feelings of men and women to being overheard whilst opening bladder or bowels.

Most people are very wrapped up in their own lives and activities and pay little attention to others. You are very sensitive and alert to your own body and its actions, but others are not, and so you may be worrying unnecessarily. You are convinced that others will hear you pass wind, smell your wet diaper, or wonder why you are spending so long in the restroom. In practice, it will be unusual for anyone else to notice. Most people pass gas from the bowel ten to twenty times per day, but how often do you hear the sound? Probably not often (unless you have a teenaged son who finds it funny or does it to annoy you)!

Dealing With Embarrassment

It is often fear of being embarrassed that leads to people with incontinence isolating themselves. If you stay at home, you do not risk being embarrassed by others seeing, hearing, or smelling your incontinence. Many people have developed strategies to avoid possibly embarrassing situations by monitoring the situation and taking preventive action to stop themselves from being let down. This "social problems prevention work" aims to alleviate embarrassment, often by helping the other person to react more positively. Remember, you only feel embarrassed due to the responses of others – if you can manage those responses in some way, you can reduce the likelihood that you will feel embarrassed. For example, you could make a comment to put others more at ease, make a joke (not always easy if you are feeling embarrassed at the time), or give a brief explanation and then move on to another topic. Sometimes, being very matter of fact about potentially embarrassing situations can relieve the tension.

Self-Esteem and Self-Confidence

We develop a sense of adult identity linked to our gender. Society has general concepts of what are masculine and feminine attributes and behaviours. If your body and behaviour will not or cannot conform to this, if you cannot be the person you feel you are or should be, or you are permanently having to pretend to be someone other than the person that you are, this can damage your self-esteem. In addition, a sense of control is important to most adults. We are mostly used to having a least some control over things in our lives. We like to be able to predict things – uncertainty is difficult to live with. Most people also feel happier if they can pinpoint a reason that something has happened to them. They can understand, for example, that they have put on weight because they have reduced the amount of exercise they do, but continue to eat the same amount of food. In the same way, people often look for a logical explanation for why they are incontinent, which means they can end up feeling in some way to blame for it:

- "If only I had done my exercises properly after childbirth"
- "If only I ate a better diet"
- "If only I could get back to a healthy weight"

If you feel that you are to blame for a situation, or that it is inevitable because of your age or an illness, then this further damages your self-esteem and this can become a vicious circle; it is difficult to motivate yourself to do something about incontinence if you really believe it cannot be improved.

It is often when people are the most desperate that they summon up the courage to ask for help; being caught out once too often by leaking urine, or having a fearful sense of bowel urgency in the midst of a crowded train carriage may be the catalyst that urges you into action. Deciding to seek help is one thing; knowing how to say what you need to say when you get there is another issue altogether.

Further Reading

This chapter has only been able to give a brief overview of what is a vast and complex subject. If you are interested in reading more, you might start with some of the books listed below. None of them is specifically dedicated to bladder and bowel function, but we hope that by understanding more about how society shapes our behaviours and reactions, you will find ways of coping with your own feelings and the reactions of others.

Green, Gill. *The End of Stigma? Changes in the Social Experience of Long-Term Illness.* London: Routledge, 2009.

Myers, Kimberly R. "Coming Out: Considering the Closet of Illness." *Journal of Medical Humanities* 25.4 (2004): 255-270.

Tangney, June Price, and Ronda L. Dearing. *Shame and Guilt.* New York: Guilford Press, 2002.

Tracy, Jessica L., Richard W. Robins, and June Price Tangney, eds. *The Self-Conscious Emotions: Theory and Research.* New York: Guilford Press, 2007.

The Boy Who Survived Incontinence

YOSHINORI KASAI, JAPAN

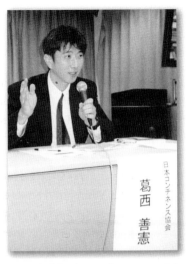

EDITOR'S NOTE: This Lived Experience was originally written in Japanese. It has been translated into English.

Prologue

I was born in Shinjuku in 1959, a time when Elvis Presley was still at his peak. While my Tokyo neighborhood displayed remarkable signs of recovery 14 years after the war, plain living was the norm. However, since conditions were the same for everyone in our neighborhood, I remember there was liveliness rather than misery there even if the living circumstances were not so affluent.

A six *tatami* mat (*tatami* are the 178 cm x 88 cm straw mats traditionally used as flooring in Japan) room served as both my father's workplace and the living space for our family. The back part of the room (partitioned off by curtains) created the space where my father worked as a masseur, while a space nearly two mats large near the entryway served as our living room. Life was not easy. My mother worked as a nurse, and as a consequence I spent long hours by myself. I think because of that I picked up techniques for how to spend time by myself. At first, it was a matter of having fun in my own world of the sort you make playing by yourself. My world in its initial form simultaneously had parts that corresponded to reality and parts for playing in my imagination, and it got so that I could change those proportions. I was able to divide my heart up into two parts partitioned by a curtain just like the single six-mat room that was our home. This would become very useful for protection later.

I remember that I used to fall a lot when I was little and I was always bruising my knees. There were also many occasions on which I came home having wet myself, but I think it didn't bother me. I also continually wet the bed, but it didn't bother me as much as it did my parents. One thing that I do remember clearly was the time I caught a cold and had diarrhea. I had developed a fever and even though I was sleeping I repeatedly soiled my underpants with watery stool. I'm certain my parents were not around that day, but an aunt who lived in the same apartment building was bothered by my repeatedly dirtying my underpants and put a diaper on me. For me, wearing diapers for the first time made me conscious of being incontinent. My aunt said, "Getting to the toilet is going to be a problem, so let's get some diapers on you." I told her "no, no" once, but I was also sluggish from the fever and gave in. I felt a sense of defeat in my later childhood over her pity and using the diaper. I think I subconsciously used the curtains in my heart to protect those parts of it that were soft.

I later learned that the cause of my incontinence was a spinal problem called spina bifida occulta. Inability to control your bladder or bowels comes with it. However, my condition was not properly diagnosed until I was 31 years old. Let me look back a little bit now at the twisting and turning path I negotiated before I knew the cause of my condition, and bring things to the present day when I know the cause and my situation has stabilized.

Elementary School Days

I traveled to my elementary school by bus. It was four stops away from my home. I wet myself to such a degree that my underpants were always soiled, but my urinary incontinence was not so bad if I went to the toilet frequently. The amount was such that I could deal with it with a towel. I noticed the smell more than the leaks themselves.

One incident left a particularly vivid impression. It happened when I was still in the lower grades of elementary school. My stomach was upset and I had diarrhea. Some stool leaked out when I was on the bus on my way to school. The situation was more a matter of my having noticed the smell of stool. I had no choice but to go back home to change my underwear and once again head for school. Class had already begun by the time I finally got to school and my homeroom teacher was very angry because I was late without having given notice. He made me stand next to the teaching platform and asked me why I was late. I was embarrassed and so I just looked down without saying anything. The teacher grew angrier at this behavior of not speaking up candidly about why I was late and hit me with his bamboo ruler. I had no choice but to give him the explanation: "I soiled myself so I went home to change my underpants." My classmates laughed, which was a great shock. My teacher then seemed to realize that he had made me say something pathetic and took pity on me. However, I was more concerned about the stares of my classmates than the teacher's supportive words. My memories of the aftermath linger in my head without a sense of reality, like images seen from a camera. It's like it was an incident seen from some other person's eyes rather than my own unpleasant memory. I think perhaps I used the curtains in my heart that I had acquired when I was little and protected myself. The curtains at that time were not a means for partitioning my heart, but rather hung over the entrance to it and kept this incident out of that opening.

I believe I was able to get through life without getting discouraged by incidents from around when I was small and easily wounded, because I was able to divide my heart in the needed proportions between fantasy and reality. In fact, even when I was in class or playing with friends I seem to have been in the world of my imagination to some extent. My nickname at the time was "Tamashii-kun" because to people around me it seemed as though my soul (*tamashii*) was not in my body at those moments when my world was more fantasy than reality. The person who gave me the name of Tamashii-kun was our homeroom teacher. I really liked that nickname.

Junior High Days

A urine test was part of the school health examinations for junior high students. Based on the results, I was examined at a hospital. The exam involved looking at my bladder by inserting a metal tube through my penis. I remember being extremely nervous sitting on the exam table. Surprisingly, the exam was painless. They said I had a urinary tract infection and prescribed antibiotics. Right when I thought I had gotten better, an incident occurred one morning – when I went to get up the futon was soaked. Furthermore, when I tried to get up, the lower half of my body was not working so well. My mother came and took me to the bathtub. My legs started to move again while I was submerged in the tub and the numbness went away. From that day forward, I would intermittently experience numbness in my legs, paralysis, and incontinence. A towel was no longer enough to deal with the blots on the futon and I found myself using diaper covers for adults with flat-type paper diapers that my mother bought at the pharmacy. The paper diapers of the day were not sufficiently absorbent because, unlike today's diapers, they did not have polymer absorbers, so they would still leak around the sides, soiling the futon and stumping us. I am filled with gratitude toward my mother, who had to shoulder a heavy burden.

My incontinence and leg paralysis symptoms continued. There was no stability. Sometimes the symptoms became more mild and sometimes more intense. Even when the symptoms were mild, the pain in my lower back and the sensation of numbness in my legs continued to recur intermittently. I would easily become constipated. Days would pass without a bowel movement if we left matters alone. Accordingly, fig enemas became part of the household medicine cabinet.

The most difficult thing about this condition was school events like field trips and school camps that involved staying somewhere. My parents would contact my homeroom teacher beforehand to explain the situation, but the problem was not one that could be solved that easily. We still had the problem of disposing of my diapers without my classmates knowing.

Unluckily, I developed problems with my appendix when it was time for our third-year field trip in junior high and I could not go. However, I was happy that being hospitalized gave me a great pretext for not being able to go.

My condition was comparatively milder during my high school and university years and I got through them with relative ease.

Work

In 1982 I got a job. Symptoms such as incontinence and paralysis continued to recur like waves. I was able to make time so that I could search with relative freedom for hospitals and folk remedies that could treat my incontinence. I was embarrassed to go to hospitals in my neighborhood, so I went knocking on the doors of countless clinics far from home. However, no matter which hospital I went to the results were not encouraging. One doctor advised me, "Incontinence is a problem involving how someone feels, so you should be firm in controlling your feelings." Another doctor, after barely examining me, said that I should practice tightening my sphincter. I also received traction and thermotherapy for my spinal cord. None of the clinics had the technology to diagnose or treat incontinence. Few hospitals in those days could conduct specialized examinations for incontinence. I think the odds of my landing at just the right hospital as I wandered blindly from one to the next were roughly the same as those for winning the lottery. The average physician did not think about trying to connect a patient to a specialized hospital for more intensive treatment since they did not judge incontinence to be a critical condition. There were few hospitals where incontinence could be treated and no network to lead you to them. Except for a fortunate few, people who suffered from incontinence could not find their way to proper treatment.

In 1984, two years after I had started working, I married a woman who joined the company the same time I did. My condition was waxing and waning as always, but at first I could not tell my bride about my incontinence. Then one day an episode of incontinence occurred in which I soaked our futon and I began to talk to her about my condition. That my wife accepted me just as she had before knowing about my control problem is a gift that I will never ever forget.

An incident that occurred at work, in which urine overflowed from my diapers, also left an impression on me. The urine ran down my chair and pooled about the floor. I was so embarrassed that I was unable to move. My co-workers cleaned the floor for me without a word. Another colleague escorted me to the toilet. I remember feeling so happy at the kindness of my co-workers.

That I had become a fully employed adult and now had financial leeway made it easier to take care of myself. For example, I could now buy the underpants-type paper diapers that I could not afford before because of their high cost. A product with polymer absorbers meant there was almost no concern about wetting the bedclothes. Also, I did not worry about bulges in my trousers even when I wore them as underwear for going outdoors because there was no need for diaper covers. Having economic resources was absolutely necessary for me to be able to continue using these costly diapers.

The Encounter

I unexpectedly came across that one thing for which I had long been searching. One day while idling at a neighborhood bookstore, the title of a book jumped out at me. It was called *Managing Incontinence*. It was such a straightforward title. The answer I had spent thirty years searching for was there in book form in front of me. The goal I had been trying and trying to reach without any success had unexpectedly appeared. I suppose that's what it means to have an encounter. I bought the book right away and hungrily searched through it. The book was from the Simon Foundation for Continence in the U.S. It contained accounts of people with incontinence, along with methods for treating it. I learned that there were physicians specializing in incontinence, various treatments for the condition, and ways of treating it yourself. However, I did not know where I could receive those treatments since the book was written in the U.S. and had been translated into Japanese, and so naturally it did not touch on such matters as who to consult in Japan.

So, taking my cue from the address at the end of the text, I wrote a letter to the Foundation. Several weeks later I received a response. The letter contained information about a hospital and physician in Nagoya with an outpatient clinic for incontinence sufferers, as well as people to consult with in Tokyo. I was introduced to a nurse named Kaoru Nishimura, who had just returned home from the U.K. after having completed her studies specializing in incontinence. I am a Tokyo resident, so I did not hesitate to call her and discuss my condition. She told me about a hospital where I could receive a diagnosis and treatment specifically for incontinence. Several weeks after this encounter with a book, I was able to go to a doctor who, like magic, was able to treat my condition.

The doctor obtained a variety of data from tests and examinations that included measuring the volume of urine I voided on my own, an ultrasound examination of my bladder, measuring how much urine remained after extracting it via a catheter, pumping carbon gas into my bladder to measure the pressure, taking X-rays and doing a CAT scan of my spinal cord, and imaging my kidneys and my bladder. The diagnosis was a neurogenic bladder due to spina bifida occulta. My condition was overflow incontinence, in which a large volume of urine remains in the bladder and eventually overflows. For me, who until then had thought that my urinary incontinence was due to my urethra not closing properly, the explanation that my condition was due to problems with voiding urine was truly a shock. The treatment method he advised me to follow was a very simple matter of voiding the urine that remained in my bladder through a tube. The quality of my life improved remarkably after I learned this self-treatment method, which is called self-catheterization. My thirty-year-long torment melted away like a piece of jigsaw puzzle settling into exactly the right spot. The road I had struggled down in my quest for the finish line measured thirty years and the distance of a letter that traveled around the world.

The Other Me

My joy over my life having become so very pleasant once learning about how to treat myself through self-catheterization was tremendous. At the same time, I was angry at the reality that the few medical institutions specializing in incontinence in Japan are so hard to find.

"The Other Me" was the phrase that crossed my mind. I sensed that there must be many people who suffer from incontinence just like I do. They should not have to experience agonies like "The Other Me." I strongly felt that I myself should get the information out. In 1993, my wife and I went to the U.S. to express my thanks to and learn about The Simon Foundation for Continence. We called upon Ms. Gartley at her home. She gave me mountains of information, and by way of thanks I taught her how to make an origami crane. I also made a promise. I promised that as long as I live, I will try to create a society in which people who suffer from incontinence will find it easier to live.

Nineteen Years Later

19 years have passed since that meeting. After coming back to Japan, I became involved with volunteer activities to support people who suffer from incontinence with whom Ms. Nishimura is working with as a health care professional. I published a book called, *Shikkin kea manyuaru* (The Incontinence Care Manual). The book's purpose is the same as that of *Managing Incontinence.*

I am thankful to have found the book, which provided the leg up that saved me.

I am thankful to all the writers of that book.

I am thankful to Ms. Nishimura, who discussed incontinence with me.

I am thankful to the physician who made the correct diagnosis.

I am thankful for the curtains in my heart.

And I am grateful to my parents and to the family that raised me and has been supportive of me.

I will continue trying to deliver my message full of love to "The Other Me" to fulfill the promise I made during that trip to America so long as I live. It would be a joy to me for this story to provide the leg up that saves you.

Stigma and You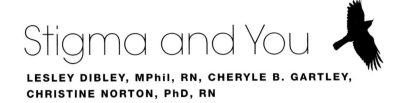

**LESLEY DIBLEY, MPhil, RN, CHERYLE B. GARTLEY,
CHRISTINE NORTON, PhD, RN**

**EDITOR'S NOTE: Incontinence is arguably one of the most stigmatized health conditions
of our time. For many individuals with incontinence there is hardly anything scarier
than the thought of having an "accident" in public. This chapter examines the consequences of being stigmatized, options for avoiding or dealing with such stigma, and
action-oriented steps that we can take to decrease the prevalence and effect of stigma.**

Stigma is a word most people struggle to define even though they may be feeling
its effects or fearing being stigma's victim. One definition of stigma, taken from
the book *The Social Psychology of Stigma,* is "1) the recognition of difference based
on some distinguishing characteristic, or 'mark'; and 2) a consequent devaluation of the
person." Stigma can be applied to various aspects of the human condition; not only to
differences of the body, but also to other categories such as "blemishes" of individual
character and differences of race, nationality, or religion. Our interest here focuses upon
the scope of the problem in healthcare and more specifically how some of the basic
components of stigma are particularly relevant to people with a misbehaving bladder
or bowel.

Anyone with a stigmatized condition will be in danger of both low self-esteem and
of being judged by others. Although you may not be able to do anything to alter the
behavior and actions of your bladder and bowel, there are things you can do to reduce
feelings of stigma, improve your self-esteem, and feel better about yourself.

Devaluation

A few of the basic components comprising stigma need to be set out as a framework
to help you fully understand its impact. One component that is especially relevant
to incontinence is the concept of discredited vs. discreditable as defined by Erving
Goffman, a sociologist who wrote the classic work on stigma. In his book *Stigma:
Notes on the Management of Spoiled Identity* Goffman refers to an important distinction

regarding people who are stigmatized due to health conditions: referring to one category as the discredited and another category as the discreditable. The difference being simply that upon first meeting a stranger their health issue is either readily apparent – for instance, someone who uses a wheelchair for mobility or a person accompanied by a guide dog (the discredited); versus meeting someone whose health challenge is not recognizable – for example, someone who has a profound hearing loss or incontinence (the discreditable).

For the discredited, life involves never being free in public, often being stared at, and constantly dealing with the public's ignorance as to how to interact with a person with a visible health condition. On the plus side, individuals in this category have the option of recognizing others in the same circumstances and entering into social interactions which might be supportive.

Individuals in the discreditable category have the ability to pass – that is, to enter society without the health challenge being known. The ability to pass is not without expense, however. It leads to various dilemmas regarding information control, such as the struggle to decide with new social contacts, or old ones for that matter, who to tell, when to tell, to lie or not to lie, and the constant awareness that at any time the choice may be taken out of your control – for instance, by having a visible episode of incontinence.

Passing

The concept of passing is a key factor if you live with incontinence, or rather, what is referred to as "social continence," which means maintaining the appearance of continence by using products to contain incontinence. Social continence, the ability of an individual to remain dry in public (often with the use of devices such as drainage systems or absorbent products), allows the individual to pass in society. However, those who choose to pass most likely live with the fear of an "accident" in public as their constant life companion. And the dilemma as to when to disclose the potentially discreditable information in intimate relationships is, for many, a prospect so daunting that they choose instead to completely ignore the opportunity for closeness in their lives.

Passing can be a very costly endeavor: it drains emotional energy, you miss the support of being open and honest with other people who may or may not have the same condition, and you give control to the public, living with the tension of not ever knowing exactly when a stranger with a curious question will "out" you.

Making the Decision to Pass or Not to Pass

There is often a fear that if you reveal that you are sometimes incontinent, others will think less of you or even reject you. Whilst this is a risk, in practice it seldom happens; we tend to select people to reveal information to when we have received some indication from them – however subtle – that they will be receptive and supportive. Revealing can also make others see you in a more positive light: the work mate who thought you were being lazy or not pulling your weight, because you were always "sneaking off" (to the toilet in fact), may now be more sympathetic and willing to cover for you as needed.

However, there is never any guarantee of how others will react, so there is always some risk to coming out about incontinence. Telling someone always carries the possibility that they in turn will tell others, so you are no longer in total control of who knows what. You must decide for yourself just how far you trust others, and how far you trust them not to spread information that you have asked them not to share. If you do find that someone responds insensitively and tactlessly to your disclosure, you may simply have to evaluate whether you really want someone who doesn't accept you and your situation in your life at all.

Another thing to keep in mind when making your decision is that others assess and make judgments about you based on what you present to them – and with no sign of whatever health challenge you might have, such as the potential for an epileptic incident, depression or incontinence, others assume you to be something different from what you are. The problem comes when you are revealed – you have a seizure, a bout of depression, or an incontinence incident and they learn of it. You are then discredited because you have shown yourself not to be the character or the person they thought you were, and their attitude and actions towards you can change as a result because they feel they have been misled.

There is no "right" or "wrong" here – you have choices and you may use different options at different times or with different people or groups. Some people may even try to keep their condition from their partner or spouse. Passing can be a more positive way of managing your feelings, because you can feel in control of who you choose to tell, and who you do not, and it is more realistic to pass when there is no benefit to be gained from coming out about your incontinence. However, passing all the time and with everybody can be an enormous physical and emotional effort because of the risk of being discovered and of having no social and emotional support network to fall back on in difficult times. Permanently passing will usually involve a lot of planning, including knowing where all the toilets are on your intended route ("toilet mapping"), taking spare supplies of products and clothes everywhere in case you need them, and endless concern and anxiety in case your body functions let you down. Even if you are very successful at disguising your incontinence from others, you may still experience incontinence as a shameful condition that damages your self-esteem.

You can learn skills of how and when to reveal information about yourself, in order to protect your well-being and to build your own social support network. Revealing, or helping others become aware of your chronic condition, can help reduce feelings of stigma. Because people are then able to know you for who you are, you need not fear discovery amongst those you have revealed to, and you cannot be discredited in their company. That openness also provides you with a support network of people who can protect you and cover for you when needed.

Controlling the information others have about you can help you feel that you are in charge of your condition, and this may help you to feel better about yourself. When you risk sharing information with others and find that their response is less critical and more supportive than you imagined, you will very likely also feel better about yourself.

Other Components of Stigma

Language and staring are major components of stigma. In the book *What Psychotherapists Should Know About Disability,* Dr. Rhoda Olkin states:

> Embedded in PC (political correctness) language are social constructs and ideologies that are important to understand. Think of the tremendous social and political changes that are implied by the terms 'girls,' 'ladies,' and 'women,' or 'colored,' 'Negro,' 'black,' and 'African American.' As we see in these examples, terminology both presages and mirrors important sociopolitical movements; it might even be argued that the changes in terminology reflect paradigm shifts.

Dr. Olkin also encourages "person first" language, stating: "Language reflects, but also creates, reality." The word "wrong" is a good example of creating reality. Individuals with stigmatized health conditions are constantly asked by complete strangers, "What is wrong with your… (fill in the body part: leg, arm, nose)?" Like multiple impressions in advertising, one wonders exactly how many times it takes for an individual with a stigmatized condition to hear the word "wrong" before that person internalizes it or takes it to heart. Person first language is the reason that in this book we refer to a person with incontinence rather than using the word incontinent as modifier (such as an "incontinent boy"). To be careful with the use of language, Goffman himself used the made-up word "Quiggle" to describe all stigmatized health conditions and thus avoid words that could accidentally stigmatize.

Unfortunately, as author Kurt Vonnegut reminds us, when we arrive on the planet we are not handed a manual entitled "Welcome to Planet Earth," with instructions included as to what to do with everything that might happen to us here. Few of us even think about stigma until we are caught in its grasp. Therefore, it is not surprising that since healthcare professionals grow up in the same culture as their patients they too are fallible to accidentally stigmatizing with words or actions. For instance, an older person ("the elderly" is considered stigmatizing in the UK) residing in a long-term care facility may feel stigmatized when a bladder diary is posted on the wall near his bed, while his doctor and nurse are completely focused on fixing the problem and totally unaware of how their behavior impacts the very person they are trying to help.

One of the challenges of a life with any type of Quiggle is that you are never sure how people are going to react if the Quiggle is known or becomes known. Being stared at is one of the fears people who are socially continent have regarding experiencing an accident in public. We are all too aware that discernable health problems so often result in a constant barrage of stares.

Additional Contributors to Stigma

The perception of cause and the fear of transmission are two reasons that health conditions are stigmatized. Some medical conditions are stigmatized because they are seen to reflect on the moral character of the person with the disease, or the illness is perceived (rightly or wrongly) to have been self-inflicted. Lung cancer, for example, may be viewed less sympathetically by onlookers who might assume – because of the proven connection between smoking and lung cancer – that the illness is self-inflicted, whilst in fact lung cancer can and does develop in those who have never smoked.

Other conditions give rise to fear that they may contaminate or be transmitted to others. Leprosy is the classic example; for centuries people with leprosy were forced to live separately from their communities (and still are in some parts of the world where leprosy still exists). HIV/AIDS, although now more accepted, still attracts negative connotations due to its perceived association with sexual or drug-injecting behavior. In these examples, and in others such as mental illness, epilepsy, and even cancer, it is fear due to lack of knowledge and understanding which causes society to respond negatively and stigmatize the condition. Incontinence is similarly perceived with prejudice by some members of society who believe it to be the "fault" of the person with incontinence.

> " *To laugh often and much; to win the respect of intelligent people and the affection of children; to earn the appreciation of honest critics and to endure the betrayal of false friends; to appreciate beauty; to find the best in others; to leave the world a bit better whether by a healthy child, a garden patch or a redeemed social condition; to know even one life has breathed easier because you have lived. This is to have succeeded.* "
>
> —Ralph Waldo Emerson

Stigma is Constantly Changing

The good news about stigma is that society continues to change its views on what is or is not a stigmatizing condition, usually in response to evidence gathered over time that the condition of interest presents less of a threat to the natural order of things than was originally thought. For example, unmarried motherhood is more accepted now than fifty years ago, but still not completely so. Similarly, in many parts of the world homosexuality is more tolerated than it was even twenty years ago, but is not universally accepted. The wide variation in the status of same-sex relationships across different states in America is evidence of this. In terms of healthcare, both cancer and AIDS have seen decreased stigma over the past few decades.

As a case in point, the September 26, 2011 USA edition of *Time* carries a full-page advertisement for a campaign entitled "Be Bold, Be Bald!" that states: "Every day, many cancer patients wonder how they're going to face the world with the symbol that everyone associates with cancer – a bald head." The campaign encourages fundraising to fight cancer by wearing a bald cap for one day, stating "It's a bold move to show your support." The advertisement features a photo of a young man with the caption: "Don't stare, I'm doing it for my brother." Images such as this would have been unimaginable just a few short years ago. Even though designed for other causes, advertisements and public relations campaigns like this one are a symbol of hope that the stigma surrounding the symptom of incontinence can also be defeated.

Academics who study stigma have also, over time, changed how they view its occurrence, now describing it as just one classification which describes life's challenges. The introduction to *The Social Psychology of Stigma* states:

> Views of the consequences of being the target of stigma have also been transformed over the past half-century. Rather than assuming that the experience of being stigmatized inevitably results in deep-seated, negative, and even pathological consequences for the personality of a stigmatized individual, researchers in this area now assume that people who are stigmatized experience a set of psychological predicaments, which they cope with using the same coping strategies as those used by non-stigmatized people when they are confronted with psychological challenges such as threats to self-esteem.

Defeating Stigma: Whose Responsibility Is It?

Psychologists Jennifer Crocker and Julie Garcia presented a paper for the Simon Foundation's 2003 *Defeating Stigma in Healthcare Conference*, which concluded:

> The great discomfort that stigmatized and non-stigmatized people feel when interacting with each is, in the final analysis, about ego. Each is afraid of being devalued, being wrong, being accused, or being inferior. These experiences are painful for our ego, but they do not represent real dangers to our well-being unless we let them. Our egos want to see us as the victim and the other person as the perpetrator. But we are all both a victim and a perpetrator when we are driven by our egos.

The solution, we have argued, lies in finding goals that are not driven by our ego. Goals about what we can learn, what relationship we want to create, or what we want to build or contribute that is larger than the self can provide the way out of the destructive cycles of interaction between the stigmatized and stigmatizer. They can help us to create trust, to find our common ground, and together to make a difference in the world.

Whether we consider stigma from the point of view of society at large, or from the reference point of how an individual can acquire new skills to cope with being stigmatized, everyone has a part to play in lessening stigma in healthcare. Regarding incontinence, for instance, each of us can help to create a culture where there is less shame around bodily functions. One way is simply by changing our vocabulary. Instead of telling children that they are "good boys" or "bad girls" depending on their success in being "potty trained," think of the difference a neutral statement such as "Isn't it nice that you are acquiring this new ability?" could make over a generation or two of use. Without the control of body functions being deemed good or bad, perhaps then adults facing changes in their ability to control a misbehaving bladder or bowel would eventually view the condition as a medical symptom to be dealt with accordingly.

Incontinence
After Prostate Cancer

ISIDORO KRASILCIC, BRAZIL

EDITOR'S NOTE: This Lived Experience was originally written in Portuguese. It has been translated into English.

I started having prostate problems when I was 49 years old. Since then I have been under medical supervision and I've had to have regular blood exams (Prostate-Specific Antigen). When I was 59, during a regular check-up, my doctor suggested a biopsy (a very difficult and painful exam) that found cancer in my prostate. The cancer was just about to reach the edge of the gland; therefore an urgent surgery was required. My PSA level was five, so I looked for a second and third opinion with two other urologists who confirmed the diagnosis.

On April 1, 2003 I had a complete prostatectomy, and afterwards I had to use a catheter for twenty days. I then had 36 radiotherapy sessions. After the radiotherapy, I started experiencing urinary incontinence. The doctor prescribed urological physiotherapy. The treatment used electrical stimulation to contract the muscle, and although embarrassing, it was very effective. The urinary incontinence improved 70% and I continued doing exercises at home.

During the first five years after this, the urinary incontinence was light, so I adapted to the situation and I became used to it. I would put on an absorbent pad in the morning that allowed me to work all day long. Then in the beginning of 2009, after urinating, I noticed some blood in the toilet. Another urologist reassured me saying that the bleeding was probably the result of the radiotherapy, but that it would be a good idea to do an exam to check the bladder internally. It was nothing serious. However, after this exam (cystoscopy with biopsy) the urinary incontinence returned much stronger. I had to replace the absorbent pads five to six times a day, in addition to the embarrassing situation of wetting my pants and underpants daily (which made me even more aggravated).

I went to see another urologist who specialized in urinary incontinence. He requested a urodynamic exam and suggested another procedure: to inject the bladder with botox. This procedure was completed, but three days after the procedure the urinary incontinence resumed at full power; therefore the procedure didn't produce any result. When the problem returned I didn't feel like working, going out, driving on the road anymore (because every time I drove my car I passed urine and it made my pants and underpants wet, and I had urine running down my leg).

Today, I am using some resources my son found on the Internet – clamps and sometimes urine collecting bags that are attached to the penis (with a collecting port and urine exit port). These devices help a lot, despite my allergy to plastic and the occasional pinching on my penis caused by the clamp (usually when I sit down or get up).

Emotionally, it was a very difficult time. First, because my sex life was over after I had such an invasive surgery. In addition, the urinary incontinence aggravated the situation even more, although I was able to adapt to these situations. Life goes on, and I have noticed that there are thousands of people with the same problems, or even worse. We should never give up because life is good. Thank God I have a wonderful family (my wife, daughter, son, son-in-law, grandkids) that give me great support, and are a reason for great pride.

I hope to find a solution for my problem soon, because I know that the medical sciences are always evolving.

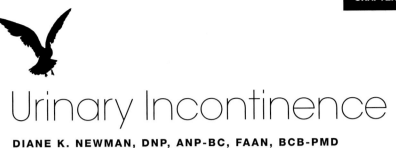

CHAPTER 3

Urinary Incontinence

DIANE K. NEWMAN, DNP, ANP-BC, FAAN, BCB-PMD

EDITOR'S NOTE: If you are experiencing any kind of urine leakage, then this chapter is for you. Urinary incontinence (UI) is also sometimes called stress incontinence, urge incontinence, overactive bladder, leaky bladder, urine leakage, loss of bladder control, or light bladder leakage. Urinary incontinence takes many forms: small occasional leaks, a sudden and uncontrollable urge to urinate, the urge to urinate frequently, or leaking urine when coughing or laughing.

Urinary incontinence (UI) is a common medical problem for both men and women. This chapter explains normal bladder and urinary tract function, causes and risk factors for UI, and the different treatment options that are available. If you are living with urinary leakage, this chapter will help you understand what is happening in your body and what you can do to treat or manage it. *Michelle has leaked urine, at least when coughing or laughing, since her last baby was born, over forty years ago. It wasn't too inconvenient... it was only a few drops each time and using a small pad was her solution. If her husband noticed that she had a problem, he never mentioned it. About five years ago, when Michelle turned seventy, she began noticing that she would get a sudden urge and would need to rush to the bathroom or lose urine on her way. She was not sure what she should do: maybe buy a larger pad?*

In 1982, Ann Landers, a well-known columnist in the United States, published a column that touched a nerve in thousands of people across the nation. Response from readers to that column was overwhelming. The subject was urinary incontinence, the involuntary leakage of urine and loss of bladder control, a condition currently affecting millions of Americans. In frank terms, the column put the problem of incontinence squarely into the public eye. That initial column was just the beginning, and over the last three decades, many columnists have highlighted urinary incontinence. 26 years later, in 2008, the daily newspaper *USA Today*, interviewed this author and her patient, Lee Greenwood, to write an insightful article titled "Incontinence: A Hidden Condition," on the impact of incontinence on a patient's life. Lee is a real estate agent who described her inability to continue in her work because of her fear of urine leakage and inability to access a bathroom while showing homes for sale. Sadly, both the Landers and *USA Today* articles noted that incontinence is such an embarrassing problem, a taboo subject for most, that it remains hidden by most sufferers.

The Problem of Urinary Incontinence

Urinary incontinence is the accidental or unwanted loss or leakage of urine, or losing urine when you don't want to. Many refer to it as "loss of bladder control," a "leaky bladder," or a "weak bladder." Incontinence episodes are often referred to as "accidents." At least one in three adult women and one in five men will experience urinary incontinence. Incontinence can vary from person to person, from day to day, and can occur rarely or frequently. The amount of urine loss can be a few drops or as much as eight ounces (240 ml).

Until recently, UI was a taboo subject, rarely disclosed by patients or openly discussed within families, and most times, undiagnosed and ignored by doctors and nurses. In addition, incontinence is an extremely costly problem for consumers and the health care industry. In terms of dollars and cents, UI annually costs the U.S. health economy $16 to $18 billion and contributes to environmental pollution. During the past decade the treatment and care of UI has undergone a revolution.

Understanding Urinary Incontinence

UI is not a normal condition nor is it a disease. Incontinence is a symptom of a bladder problem or the result of side effects of medications or an illness. A chronic medical problem, it can disable even a young person. It is feared by those who suffer with it, unrecognized by many medical professionals, and generally misunderstood by the public. Health care professionals estimate that UI affects more Americans than any other medical problem, condition, or disease. It is the second major cause of an older person being admitted to a nursing home.

Despite its prevalence, women wait an average of three-and-a-half years years before seeking help. An Internet study by this author indicated that more than half of women who discussed overactive bladder (OAB), an incontinence-related condition, with a health care provider waited longer than one year to seek treatment. Other surveys show that a woman may view unwanted leakage of urine as part of being a woman, just another nuisance to deal with. Being incontinent is embarrassing and is not a subject for polite conversation. More unfortunately, it is not even a subject at most patient-doctor interviews. Doctors have an attitude of "don't ask and don't tell." In the case of female patients, doctors, inattentive to the special health needs of women, do not recognize UI as a unique medical condition. As a result, they do not diagnose it. Older patients are reluctant to mention their condition to doctors and nurses because they believe that it is just the natural result of aging. Even some doctors and nurses view UI as an "old age" condition. Other patients, lacking knowledge about both the functioning of their bodies and misunderstanding what incontinence is, believe there is no treatment for incontinence and there is no use bothering the doctors and nurses about it. Instead, they either ignore their problem, on the theory that it will resolve itself, or they substitute incontinence products for medical help. They "self-manage" their incontinence.

Many people go to great lengths to hide their problem. They can't, or believe they can't, tell others about their problem without receiving pity or disgust from those closest to them. They don't visit with friends because they can't sit long enough to play one hand of bridge without needing to void. They are uncomfortable at parties and dinners, fretting that an odor of urine surrounds their clothes and bodies. When they wear incontinence products, they have the constant fear that urine will leak onto outer garments and furniture. Some wash underclothes and sheets by hand to hide urine stains from the people who do their laundry. Others worry that there won't be a place to change their clothing should an accident occur. Some rarely attend church services, others give up movies or the theater, and many avoid long trips and travel. Sleep deprivation is also common among people with incontinence, who wake themselves up several times during a night to make trips to the bathroom. Even long-standing relationships are broken, sometimes never to be mended again. The consequences of an incontinence problem creep into every part of their lives.

Urinary incontinence is a burden for persons who experience it, but also has a dramatic impact on the lives of families, friends, and caregivers. Many people with UI become depressed and, in time, develop severe psychological and physiological problems. Dealing with an incontinent, depressed parent or mate puts a strain on family relationships. Sufferers with physical limitations, such as walking difficulties or mental impairment, need special care. The family has a difficult time dealing with a stubborn, uncooperative individual who may have a negative attitude toward a UI problem. Additionally, availability and kind of care, along with economic concerns play a large role in a family's ability to cope with incontinence and a relative with incontinence. These problems place pressure on the time and type of care and attention a family can expend.

Normal Bladder Function

Emily's bladder has always been in control. Over the years, she has learned the location of every restroom at the malls and in many cases will not go to unfamiliar places. Before driving from her house to see her daughter, she always uses the bathroom, even if she doesn't need to. Emily feels she has "weak" kidneys; her doctor told her she has a weak bladder. Emily, like most people, doesn't understand how her bladder works. To understand why you may have an incontinence problem, you need to under-stand bladder control or continence. Normal functioning of the lower urinary tract, the bladder, urethra, and urinary sphincters is necessary, as is pelvic floor muscle support.

The Parts of the Lower Urinary Tract

Urination (voiding) or "passing your water" is controlled by your lower urinary tract, which includes the bladder, the urethra, the sphincters, and the muscles that surround the urethra and sphincters. This is often called the "pelvic area." The following illustration shows this area.

Figure 1. Male and female pelvic areas

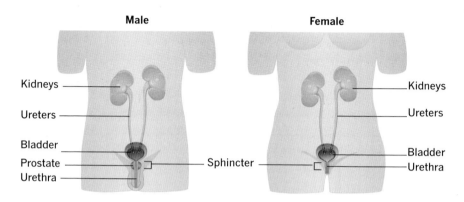

The bladder is a muscle and tissue that stores or "holds" urine produced by the kidneys. The bladder is sometimes referred to as the "detrusor." The bladder is located in the pelvis behind the pelvic bone. It changes shape when there is more or less urine in it. When empty, it resembles a deflated balloon or is flat as a pancake. As it fills with urine, its shape looks like a football. The urethra is a small, slender tube that starts at the bottom or base of the bladder (called the bladder neck) and goes to the outside of the body. In women the urethra is about one-and-a-half inches long. The vagina is behind the urethra. The opening of the urethra is called the urethral meatus and is located between the clitoris and the vaginal opening (see the following figure). Because the clitoris, vaginal opening, and urethra are located so close to each other in a very small area, the urethra is not easy to find. A woman may need to use a mirror to help locate her urethra.

Figure 2. Female genital area

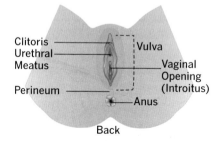

In men the urethra is around eight inches long. It leaves the bladder, passes through the prostate gland, the pelvic muscle, and the length of the penis, ending at the opening at the tip or glans of the penis. The prostate is a walnut-sized gland located at the base of the bladder. It surrounds the urethra like a doughnut. The portion closer to the urethra can enlarge, causing obstruction which can prevent the man from completely emptying his bladder. A common condition seen in men as they age is BPH, enlargement of the prostate gland. BPH can cause an obstruction or narrowing of the urethra, leading to symptoms of urgency and frequency and, in some cases, incontinence. The main function of the prostate is the manufacture of secretions that become components of semen.

Regulation of the storage and emptying of urine from the bladder is controlled by the internal and external urinary sphincters. A sphincter is a ring-like band of muscle fibers that closes off natural body openings, such as the anus and the urethra. The internal sphincter is at the bottom or base of the bladder and the external one is below it and surrounding the urethra. These sphincters are like "valves" as they keep the bladder from emptying and close the urethra until you want to void. They are supposed to stay tight or closed without a person needing to think about it. When sitting, standing, or walking, urine does not leak out of the bladder or urethra because the sphincters maintain closure of the urethra. The sphincters relax and open when nerves from your brain and spinal cord tell you to empty your bladder.

Pelvic Floor Muscles

The pelvic floor muscles are a group of muscles that go from the front (anterior) to the back (posterior) of the pelvis around the rectum, forming a sling that supports the organs of the lower urinary tract. This muscle is sometimes referred to as the pubococcygeus or levator ani muscle. The pelvic floor is not a rigid platform, but a strong, flexible muscular structure, often described as a hammock. The pelvic floor muscle has striated muscle fibers which are under voluntary control (under your control) and can be exercised. The pelvic floor surrounds, suspends, and anchors the pelvic organs, helping them remain in place. These muscles contract and expand during voiding and bowel movements. In men, the pelvic muscle surrounds the prostate and external urinary sphincter.

Figure 3. Male and female pelvic floor muscles

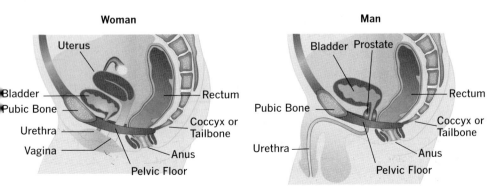

Normal bladder function in both men and women is difficult to maintain without the strength and support of the pelvic floor muscles. In women, these muscles can be used during sexual intercourse for the stimulation of a partner's penis. When infection or physical trauma damages the pelvic floor, the tone, or firmness, and health of pelvic muscles and nerves are affected, causing pelvic organs in women—the bladder neck (i.e., lower part of the bladder), urethra, or the uterus—to drop or sag (called pelvic organ prolapse).

The Brain and Nervous System

In simple terms, continence and incontinence is really controlled by your brain, spinal cord, and nerves. Parts of your nervous system are located in your brain and along your spinal cord, as well as the nerves in your bladder and the sphincters. Bladder function involves involuntary and voluntary muscle systems and a complex combination of nervous system components.

Continence or incontinence is controlled by messages exchanged between your brain and your muscle and nervous system. As an infant, a person has little control over the urge to void. As the brain, muscles, and nerves mature, a "Bladder Control Central" develops. Located in the base of the brain, the Bladder Control Central coordinates sphincter relaxation during voiding. Urinary continence results when each system receives and correctly responds to the messages. Incontinence results when there is a breakdown in communication between the Bladder Control Central, the bladder, and the sphincter. This breakdown may be caused by a mental or a physical impairment or by a disease like stroke, Parkinson's disease, or multiple sclerosis. If the nerves to the bladder no longer work, then a person may develop a "neurogenic" bladder or neurogenic bladder overactivity and experience UI, urgency, frequency, and incomplete bladder emptying.

Figure 4. The urinary system

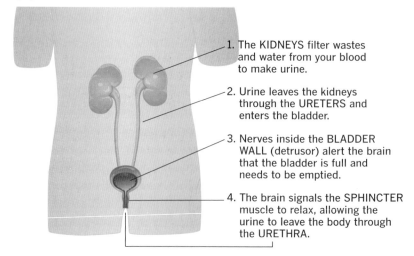

1. The KIDNEYS filter wastes and water from your blood to make urine.

2. Urine leaves the kidneys through the URETERS and enters the bladder.

3. Nerves inside the BLADDER WALL (detrusor) alert the brain that the bladder is full and needs to be emptied.

4. The brain signals the SPHINCTER muscle to relax, allowing the urine to leave the body through the URETHRA.

Voiding or "Passing Your Water"

The voiding (urinating) cycle has two phases: the bladder-filling phase and the emptying or voiding phase. Normally, the bladder muscle is relaxed while it fills with urine. When the bladder is full, a signal is sent to the brain that creates an urge to void. This is different from "urgency" (a sudden strong desire to urinate that is hard—or impossible—to delay). When a person feels that voiding is appropriate (the right place and time), he or she relaxes the urinary sphincter, the bladder muscle contracts, and the flow of urine begins.

The Path to Normal Voiding

The lower urinary tract is essentially a high-volume, low-pressure system. As long as the pressure within the urethra remains higher than the pressure within the cavity of the bladder, you will be continent or dry. Even when the bladder is full, it is elastic enough to accommodate additional fluid without causing pressure within the bladder. The bladder holds between 12 and 15 ounces (360 to 450 ml) of urine. Normally you will feel the urge to void when the bladder contains about eight to ten ounces of urine, about as much fluid as in a can of soda. There really are no "normal" voiding patterns. Normal can range from every four to six hours to every six to eight hours. Seniors over 65 may void every three to four hours and at least once during the night. The urge to void is a sensation or feeling that makes you want to empty your bladder. Usually it indicates your bladder is full. However, if you have frequent voiding and incontinence, the bladder may not be full, but may be contracting and producing urgency.

Helping Your Bladder to Empty

Problems with bladder control or incontinence may be caused by conditions that keep the bladder from emptying completely (e.g., diabetes, multiple sclerosis, stroke). When voiding occurs, some urine may stay in the bladder. This remaining urine can cause you to feel more urgency and the need to void more often. Not fully emptying your bladder can also increase your risk of a urinary tract or bladder infection, so always empty your bladder in a relaxed and private place. Worry and tension can make bladder emptying harder. Women should sit comfortably on the toilet seat and relax the pelvic floor muscle to void. Men can stand, but if it seems hard to void fully when standing, then they should sit. Do not push down on your bladder with your hands or stomach to help urinate.

What You Can Do to Urinate More Completely

Here are ways to help you empty your bladder more completely:

- change the position of your upper body by rocking or leaning forward on the toilet, or
- once you have stopped voiding, stand up, sit back down, lean forward, and try to void again, or
- when voiding stops, wait on the toilet for three to five minutes and then exhale through your mouth only, as if you are blowing through a straw. Then try voiding.

If you have a hard time relaxing to void, you can try other methods to trigger the bladder to contract, such as placing your hands in warm water, listening to running water, or pouring water over your groin, penis, or outside the vagina or pubic area.

Bladder Changes with Aging

Amelia had just turned 78 and was starting to feel old. She found herself going to the bathroom once an hour and getting up twice at night to void. Sometimes the "urge" came on so quickly that she was afraid she wouldn't get there if she didn't make a run for it. Many times she put paper towels between her legs just in case she had an accident. When she told her family doctor about the problem, he just shook his head and cautioned her to be careful not to fall when she was rushing to the bathroom. Bladder sensation changes with age, and Amelia describes many of those changes. Seniors, instead of perceiving the bladder filling at half-capacity as younger people do, may feel the need to void only when the bladder is almost full. To an active, mobile person, no matter what age, locating toilet facilities may be an inconvenience. To an immobile adult, a senior citizen, or an individual with an unstable bladder, "warning time," the time between the realization of the need to void and the actual release of urine, is critical. Delaying voiding can result in urinary incontinence.

> " *The longer I live, the more I realize the impact of attitude on life. Attitude to me is more important than facts. It is more important than the past, than education, than money, than circumstances, than failures, than success, than what other people think or say or do. It is more important than appearance, gift, or skill … .* "
>
> — *Charles Swindoll*

Another age-related change is that bladder capacity is diminished. The bladder muscle shrinks in size or capacity and cannot hold as much urine as it did in younger years. Therefore, seniors get the urge to void with lower bladder volumes and urgency may be more intense and occur suddenly.

Seniors produce their greatest volume of urine at night, two-thirds of their daily fluid intake is excreted at night. This is because older adults tend to have more medical problems such as hypertension and heart problems, and the heart is not as efficient at pumping all the fluid during daytime activity. By the end of the day, many persons will notice edema or "swelling" in their ankles and feet. So during the night when you are lying flat and at rest, the heart is able to more efficiently pump the extra fluid and the kidneys are able to filter wastes and produce urine more efficiently, leading to larger nighttime voided volumes (called "nocturnal polyuria"). Seniors may need to use the bathroom one or more times a night (called "nocturia"). Seniors who do not completely empty their bladders make many trips to the bathroom during a night.

Causes of Urinary Incontinence

There are two main types of urinary incontinence: stress or urgency. In young adults each can occur alone, but older adults and seniors often suffer from a combination of stress and urgency urinary incontinence called mixed urinary incontinence.

Urgency urinary incontinence is the involuntary leakage of urine accompanied by or immediately preceded by urgency. Involuntary or "overactive" bladder contractions cause the pressure in the bladder to exceed pressure in the urethra sufficiently to cause urine loss. This condition is referred to as "overactive bladder," or OAB, and includes symptoms of urgency, a sudden and usually uncontrollable need to urinate, and frequency, which is going to the bathroom more than eight times a day. The amount of urine loss may be large (greater than 100 ml or three ounces), and the bladder may not empty completely. Persons with urgency incontinence will complain that the urine just "gushes" out. A common sequence of urgency, often referred to as "key in the lock" or "garage door syndrome," is strong urges to void as soon as one returns home, regardless of how recently the bladder was emptied. The person is very aware of the need to urinate and yet can't seem to get to the toilet before having an accident.

When UI occurs at night, it is called "nocturnal enuresis" or "bedwetting." In many cases, these symptoms are related to overactivity of the bladder, but they can also be caused by other forms of bladder dysfunction. Also, certain activities or events may "trigger" sudden urgency and urine leakage. Some common ones include hearing running water, washing dishes or clothes, placing your hands in warm water, anxiety or stressful situations, and exposure to cold (e.g., leaving a warm house to go out into the cold). Another symptom of urgency incontinence is called "frequency," which is voiding more than eight times during the day and night. You may feel you void too often. Usually your sleep is disturbed because you have to awaken at night one or more times due to the need or urge to void. Of the three symptoms: urgency, frequency and urge UI, frequency is most commonly reported in persons with overactive bladder, and urgency urinary incontinence the least common.

The second type of urinary incontinence is called **stress urinary incontinence.** This has nothing to do with mental stress, but is all about stress or pressure on the bladder which causes a small amount of urine leakage with physical exertion or activity. As the stress, or pressure, increases, the bladder can't handle it, because the pelvic support network isn't strong enough. Laughing, coughing, sneezing, running, jumping, exercising, lifting, sitting, standing, and other strenuous physical activities cause a rise in abdominal pressure leading to stress incontinence. These activities increase pressure on your abdomen, causing pressure on your bladder. Another complaint you may have is losing urine when getting up from a chair because your abdominal muscles push down on your bladder, causing urine leakage. This type of incontinence usually produces only small amounts or "drops" of urine leakage. However, the amount of leakage may change, depending on the specific activities that cause the urine loss and how severe your sphincter problem happens to be. Severe stress incontinence can even occur during minimal activity, such as changing positions in bed, or the leakage may not be related to any activity. Causes include weakened muscles in the pelvic floor, which cause the bladder and urethra to sag or shift downwards. Stress incontinence in men can be caused by prostate surgery, especially for cancer, which can damage the urethral sphincter muscle.

Who Is at Risk?

Incontinence is not an ordinary and inevitable part of the aging process and it is also not part of being female. Many factors contribute to an incontinent condition as it is seen in women and men of all ages and occurs in many areas of daily life. Pregnancy and childbirth, prostate surgery, loss of estrogen after menopause, physical and mental disabilities, medication, and surgery may all contribute to the loss of pelvic floor muscle tone and nerve damage. Here is a review of the risks associated with UI:

- **Pregnancy and childbirth** can influence urinary control in some women. It is not uncommon for women who have previously had normal control to start having accidents while they are pregnant. Half of all women pregnant for the first time experience bladder control problems that start during the first trimester. Bladder control problems may become more severe with each additional pregnancy. The strain of childbirth, vaginal delivery, and an episiotomy, a procedure that involves cutting into the pelvic floor muscles, weaken pelvic floor structures. The incontinence may persist after childbirth.
- **High-impact exercises** like running and high-impact aerobics (especially jumping with legs apart) result in more episodes of incontinence than do other sports. High-impact movements subject the pelvic floor to forces three to four times a woman's body weight, and pelvic floor ligaments cannot sustain these high forces for prolonged periods. They also cause further damage, especially if a woman already has weak pelvic muscles. The amount of urine loss depends on the mechanical pressure. This may explain why young women who have never been pregnant become incontinent during sports. Low-impact activities in which one foot is always on the floor may allow many women to exercise without urine loss.
- **Loss of the estrogen hormone** in women after menopause may cause thinning of the tissues surrounding and supporting the pelvic organs, including the bladder, and incontinence may result.
- **Enlargement of the prostate gland** in men may prevent the bladder from emptying completely, and urine can leak or dribble out. If a man ignores symptoms of urgency and frequency, which may be the result of an enlarged prostate, it can lead to the bladder decompensating, causing incontinence.
- **Urinary tract infections** occur more frequently in women as they grow older, and can predispose some to urgency and frequency.

- **Chronic medical conditions** such as diabetes, stroke, and multiple sclerosis may result in UI and OAB symptoms of urgency and frequency. Medical conditions, Alzheimer's, Parkinson's, and dementia may impair a person's mental ability. Communication lines between the brain and the bladder get crossed and continence messages are not received by the nerves to the bladder and pelvis. These conditions can lead to a neurogenic bladder.

- **Multiple medications** may further predispose individuals to urinary symptoms. When medication is not carefully prescribed and monitored, not only UI, but mental confusion and serious health complications may be the result. Medications that can negatively affect the bladder include blood pressure drugs, cold remedies (e.g., antihistamines), diuretics (water pills), antidepressants, pain medications, and sleeping pills.

- **Visual and mobility changes** may impair an individual's ability to get to a toilet before urinary leakage occurs. Persons who have mobility or balance problems may be unable to suppress an urge to urinate until a caregiver arrives to toilet them. Many individuals who use assistive devices, such as canes, walkers, and a wheelchair, have a difficult time accessing toilet facilities; they may be unable to walk or propel their wheelchairs to the toilet in a timely fashion. These individuals benefit from convenient bathroom facilities and bedside commodes, sufficient lighting, and special bathroom fixtures, such as railings, low toilets, or adapted toilet seats.

Assessment of Urinary Incontinence

Finding a cause for your incontinence is the first and most important part of the evaluation and treatment of UI, and this assessment can be performed by your family doctor. Writing down your symptoms, problems, and questions before visiting your doctor is a good idea. This allows you to think about your problem before your visit. Answering the most commonly asked questions before seeing someone allows you more time to think about your answers so that you thoroughly understand your incontinence. So ask yourself the following questions and write down your answers:

- Do you get a sudden feeling that you need go to the bathroom immediately and you cannot ignore it? (urgency)
- Do you experience a loss of urine when you sneeze, cough, or laugh? (stress incontinence)
- Do you sometimes experience urine leakage on the way to the bathroom? (urgency incontinence)
- How often do you go to the bathroom? Is it more than eight times in a 24-hour period? (frequency)
- Do you get up at night to go to the bathroom? If so, how often? Does the urge to urinate wake you up? (nocturia)
- When you have the urge to urinate, do you sometimes have wetting accidents?
- Do you avoid going to places if you do not know the location of the restroom?
- Do you use pantiliners or pads in your underwear to keep from wetting your clothes?

Figure 5. Bladder Diary

Time	Amount Voided (Ounces or mls)	Urine Leakage	Reason for Urine Leakage or Voiding (Urgency, coughing, bending)	Amount and Type of Fluid Intake
1:00 am	5 oz		Woke up, went to toilet	4 oz water
3:00 am	4 oz		Woke up, went to toilet	
5:30 am	5 oz	√	Urgency, rushing to toilet	3 oz water
7:00 am				8 oz coffee, 6 oz milk
7:30 am	4 oz	√	Showering, urgency	
10:30 am				6 oz coffee, 4 oz water
12:00 pm	4 oz		Slight urgency	
1:30 pm		√		7 oz water, 16 oz diet soda
2:00 pm	7 oz		Strong urge	
3:15 pm	5 oz			4 oz energy drink
5:00 pm	6 oz	√	Leak with a sneeze	
6:00 pm				4 oz water, 8 oz diet soda, 4 oz glass wine
8:15 pm	7 oz		Urgency	
9:30 pm	6 oz			

Circle the product you are using

 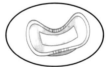

Pantiliner   Pads   Underwear   Brief or Diaper

Number of products you used today ___4___

As part of determining the history and specifics of your incontinence, you may be asked to provide a "picture" of your problem by keeping a Bladder Diary (see Figure 5) of your voiding patterns, diet habits, and UI episodes. Each column requests specific information that provides information about your individual symptoms.

Column 1 – Write the time of day or night when you void, had an incontinent episode, or drank something.

Column 2 – Measure the amount of urine you void, because this can give a picture of the amount of urine your bladder is holding.

Column 3 – Note each time you leak urine or have an accident.

Column 4 – Describe the activity you were doing when the accident occurred, such as due to a sudden urgency, on the way to the bathroom, laughing.

Column 5 – Note the type of liquid intake (e.g., coffee, water, etc.) and estimate the amount (e.g., one cup) you drank.

On the bottom of the record, if you use any pads for protection, circle the type and write in the number.

As part of evaluating your incontinence, you will need to have an examination that includes your abdomen, pelvis, rectum, and nervous system. A general examination to detect conditions such as edema—swelling in your legs, ankles, and feet—will also be done. Your urine will be checked for infection and a portable ultrasound may be necessary to see if you are able to completely empty your bladder.

Treatments

In most cases urinary incontinence can be treated or managed successfully, but most people are unaware of what is available. The solution for UI involves lifestyle changes, exercises, retraining the bladder, drug therapy, and in certain cases surgery.

Medications

Usual drug therapy for urgency incontinence consists of drugs that decrease unwanted bladder contractions or bladder overactivity. They are called antimuscarinic and anticholinergic medications (such as darifenacin, fesoterodine, oxybutynin [oral and in patch or gel form], tolterodine, solifenacin, trospium), and can help you if you are experiencing symptoms of urgency incontinence, urgency and/or frequency. These drugs act by preventing the release of a chemical called acetylcholine, from receptors in the bladder. Acetylcholine causes the bladder to contract. These drugs work in about two to three weeks. Because the same receptors that are in the bladder are also found throughout the body, in the brain, eye, nasal and salivary glands, and gastrointestinal system, some side effects occur in these other organs. Some people experience dry mouth and constipation and, rarely, more serious side effects such as blurred vision and urinary retention (inability to pass urine or empty the bladder completely). These drugs should not be taken if you have urinary retention, gastric retention, or uncontrolled narrow-angle glaucoma. There is a drug for stress incontinence called duloxetine, but it is not approved in the United States for use in persons with incontinence.

Behavioral Treatments

The best way to learn new behavior or to relearn old behavior is by identifying the desired behavior and gradually outlining the steps to be taken to achieve the desired behavior. This shaping or outlining is achieved through goal setting and positive reinforcement if goals are achieved. A very successful UI treatment is behavioral treatment or conservative therapies. There are treatments you can do on your own. An important part of any behavioral treatment program is the monitoring of voiding patterns and specified behavior. This is accomplished through the use of a Bladder Diary (see page 38). A critical part of any behavioral program is the feedback from the clinician or caregiver in settings such as nursing homes or in-home care. There are several different behavioral treatments, including self-care or lifestyle practices, bladder training programs, and pelvic floor muscle exercises. Specific treatments depend on the individual's motivation and mental capabilities.

Lifestyle or Self-Care Practices

Lifestyle changes such as modifying diet, regulating fluid intake, avoiding constipation, losing weight, monitoring medications, and smoking cessation can all improve UI symptoms.

- **Stop smoking** – Nicotine in cigarettes can be irritating to the bladder muscle, causing overactive bladder symptoms of urgency. Also, a smoker's repeated and chronic coughing may cause stress urinary incontinence, and smoking cessation may help to decrease urine leakage.
- **Maintain a healthy weight** – Being overweight can put pressure on your bladder, which may cause leakage of urine when you laugh or cough. If you are overweight, losing some weight can lessen the pressure on your bladder, as even a small amount of weight loss, maybe 5 – 10%, can make a difference.
- **Modify fluid intake** – Individuals with urinary symptoms often limit fluids so that they will not have to urinate as often. Unless your doctor or nurse tells you to, don't stop drinking water and juice because of being afraid of wetting yourself. A smaller amount of urine in the bladder leads to more concentrated (darker) urine that can cause urinary urgency, frequency, and urine leakage. So drink water every day, just do not drink large amounts at one time. Individuals with urgency incontinence who drink large amounts of fluids (>2,400 ml/day), may have fewer incontinent episodes and urinate less often by not drinking as much. Drinking too much fluid will cause you to go to the bathroom more often. You should avoid extremes in the amount you drink (neither too much nor too little). You should "drink to your thirst," and your urine should be pale yellow. Try not to drink large amounts at one time; instead, sip two to

three ounces every twenty to thirty minutes between meals. It is unlikely that you will need to drink more than one-and-a-half quarts (eight cups or 1,500 ml) of total fluids each day.

- **Check your diet for bladder irritants** – Certain food and beverages can irritate the bladder and make symptoms worse. Their effect on the bladder is not always understood, and the same food or beverage may affect different people in different ways. Persons who have problems with frequent urination and urinary incontinence are advised to decrease or eliminate alcohol, sweetener substitutes or diet beverages that contain aspartame, and caffeinated drinks and foods from their diets. Think about what you eat. Check this list of foods and drinks to see if any of them are adding to your symptoms. You may want to stop eating these foods for two weeks to see if your bladder symptoms improve. Then introduce them one at a time to see if you notice any changes.

  - **Caffeine** is found naturally in coffee beans, tea leaves, and cocoa beans. More than 80% of the U.S. adult population consumes caffeine (at least 200 mg/day) on a daily basis in the form of coffee, tea, or soft drinks. A twelve-ounce cup of brewed coffee contains 200 mg of caffeine. Tea has approximately 30 – 50 mg of caffeine for each eight-ounce serving. Herbal teas may contain caffeine unless the label indicates otherwise (e.g., says caffeine-free). Sodas (e.g., Mountain Dew, Pepsi, Coca-Cola) and candy that contain milk chocolate have caffeine. Avoid too much caffeine intake (e.g., no more than 200 mg per day or no more than two cups of caffeinated drinks per day), but cut down on caffeine slowly to avoid withdrawal symptoms (e.g., migraine-type headache).

  - **Alcohol** – beer, wine, hard liquor – causes your kidneys to produce more urine which quickly fills the bladder, causing frequent urination.

  - **Other foods** that may irritate the bladder include citrus juices and fruits, highly spiced foods, milk/milk products, carbonated beverages, sugar, honey, and corn syrup. Experiment to see which one may be affecting your bladder and causing your symptoms and if you suspect one of them is the cause, then eliminate it from your diet to see if your symptoms improve.

- **Herbs that affect the bladder** contain active ingredients that work on our bodies. There is very little research on the effects of herbs, but the ones in the list on the following page are said by some to affect bladder and bowel function.

> " *If you celebrate your differentness, the world will, too. It believes exactly what you tell it——through the words you use to describe yourself, the actions you take to care for yourself, and the choices you make to express yourself. Tell the world you are one-of-a-kind creation who came here to experience wonder and spread joy. Expect to be accommodated.* "
>
> — *Victoria Moran*

Herb	Effect
Cornsilk	May make tissues of the bladder stronger. Is very mild and nontoxic. It may help lessen urine leakage and bedwetting.
Parsley	Has a diuretic effect (i.e., increases the amount of urine produced) by preventing the body from absorbing salt.
Buchu leaf	Acts on the kidneys by increasing the amount of urine produced and ridding the body of wastes. A combination of concentrated cranberry juice and Buchu leaf is used as a diuretic.
Uva ursi leaf	The main ingredient, arbutin, can disinfect the urine, especially if the urine is alkaline. Can also be a strong diuretic.
Rhubarb	Is a mild laxative that produces a soft bowel movement in about six to ten hours. A side effect may be stomach cramping.
Cascara	Dried and cured, it is one of the most effective, gentle, and non-habit-forming laxatives. It will produce a soft or formed bowel movement in about six to eight hours.
Ginger root	Good laxative if you have constipation.
Irish moss	A bulk laxative in its raw form, it coats and soothes the entire GI tract.
Slippery elm	Helps control diarrhea by absorbing toxins from the bowel; also regulates intestinal flora (naturally occurring bacteria) while soothing the lining of your bowels.

- **Minimize nighttime voiding** – Awakening at night to void or incontinence while asleep (called nocturnal enuresis or bedwetting) can be particular problems for both the individual and the caregiver, especially if family members must get up to assist with toileting. Efforts should be made to maximize the sleep period as patterns change with age and sleep becomes fragmented. There is a decreased amount of deep sleep (Stages 3 and 4) and higher percentage of Stage 1 sleep. Therefore, sleep occurs for shorter periods with many awakenings. The following strategies may help:
  - Reduce what you drink in the evening, after around 6 pm. Concentrate on drinking more of your liquids during morning and afternoon hours to decrease the number of voiding and incontinence episodes during the night. If you have to take pills at bedtime, take them with only a small amount of water.
  - Always urinate before going to bed.
  - Increase urine output during the day by taking a one to two hour nap or rest with legs elevated to level of your heart. If you increase urine output during the day, you may decrease output and the number of voids during the night.
  - Wear support stockings during the day if you have swelling in your legs.
  - If you take a diuretic, change the time you take it, take it at two in the afternoon instead of in the early morning. But check with you doctor first.

- **Check the medications you are taking** – Some over-the-counter medications (e.g., drugs for headaches or menstrual cramps) contain caffeine, which can worsen bladder problems.
- **Keep your bowels regular** – Keeping healthy bowel habits may lessen bladder symptoms. Soft, regular bowel movements can lessen urgency and help prevent urine leakage. Constipation and difficulty with defecation (straining during bowel movements) can put more pressure on the bladder, causing urgency and urine leakage. Straining and pushing down to have a bowel movement can weaken the pelvic muscles. Some suggestions to keep bowels soft and regular include: 1) increasing fiber-rich foods in your diet such as beans, oatmeal, bran cereal, whole wheat bread and pasta, fresh fruits and vegetables; 2) exercising daily to promote regular bowel movements; and 3) drinking plenty of nonirritating fluids (water). See Chapter 4 for more details on bowel problems.

Pelvic Floor Muscle Exercises

Pelvic floor muscle exercises and training can decrease urine leakage associated with a weak pelvic floor muscle. Contracting the pelvic floor muscle provides support, lengthens and compresses the urethra, and maintains the angle between the bladder and urethra in its proper position. A strong pelvic floor muscle decreases the problem of frequent urination and the feeling of urgency to urinate. Actively exercising this muscle usually improves urinary control. The goal of pelvic floor muscle training is to find your muscle and exercise it to make it stronger and thicker. Then you use it to prevent urgency and incontinence. It is important to correctly find your muscle. When women contract their pelvic floor muscle when sitting, they will feel a slight pulling in the anus and vagina. When contracting the muscle, men will feel a pulling in the anus and movement of the penis. One way to correctly contract the muscle is to squeeze the back part of the pelvic floor muscle that surrounds your anus to prevent the passing of gas (wind). If you feel a "pulling" sensation at the anus, you are using the right muscles. Repeating pelvic floor muscle exercises on a regular basis increases the force and duration of muscle contractions. The exercises involve two types of contractions:

- **Quick (Flicks)** – Tighten and relax the pelvic muscle as rapidly as possible. Avoid bearing down or straining and contracting your stomach, thighs, or buttocks.
- **Slow** – Tighten the pelvic muscle, hold for a count of five, then relax. Direct the force of your contraction inward and upward.

It is recommended that you perform at least thirty exercises twice a day. Bladder symptoms usually improve within one month after starting the exercises, but by three to six months, you should see significant changes. But symptoms improve slowly and tracking symptom improvement is essential. Also, check with your doctor or nurse to make sure you are doing these exercises correctly, and also perhaps check again; so many people give up because their symptoms don't improve, and they haven't even done the exercise correctly to begin with. A daily Bladder Diary is an excellent way to mark progress and point out the success of the exercises.

Bladder Training Programs

There are several bladder training programs that are part of behavioral treatments that help a person to become continent or to lessen incontinence episodes and bladder symptoms. The first is bladder training that requires a person to resist the sensation of urgency, to postpone voiding, and to urinate by the clock, rather than in response to urgency. The person uses strategies called "urge suppression" to decrease frequent voids and to decrease urgency that may lead to incontinence. Here is an example of these strategies:

Carolyn has had problems with leaking urine while rushing to the bathroom. She rushes because of strong urges she cannot control. The nurse practitioner at her doctor's office gave her some "tricks" to try so she wouldn't leak. So now when she watches TV and gets a strong urge to urinate, she stops before getting up out of the chair to walk to the bathroom, and takes some slow deep breaths to relax her bladder. She waits a few minutes, then gets up and goes to urinate. She no longer rushes to the bathroom as she knows she is going to get there in time as the urgency is not as strong! She has also tried this when she feels urgency when unlocking the front door to her apartment. She will just stop, relax, and take some slow, deep breaths or do a few quick pelvic muscle squeezes until the urge lessens or passes. Then, she unlocks the door and walks slowly to the toilet.

The goal for Carolyn is to improve bladder overactivity by learning techniques that can control urgency and decrease frequency. This will hopefully increase bladder capacity and reduce urgency incontinence episodes. An important part of bladder training is education about continence as a learned behavior and the importance of the brain's control over lower urinary tract function. A scheduling regimen is an essential component of bladder training. As part of this program, you will need to increase time between voids by ten to fifteen minutes every couple of days to weekly. For example, if you are voiding every thirty minutes, then you will need to wait 45 minutes before voiding. Once you are able to wait 45 minutes, then increase to one hour. Ideally, by the end of four to six weeks, you will be able to wait two to four hours to void.

As Carolyn in the example above learned, another essential part of bladder training is education on ways to increase bladder control by delaying voiding and practicing distraction strategies. Concentration on a task requiring close attention is useful in distracting the individual from the sensation of urgency. Learning to relax can lessen your strong urge feeling and allow you to wait longer before using the bathroom. You will then stop the habit of frequent voiding, improve your ability to stop urine leakage, and cut down on urinary urgency. You may think that the only way to relieve your feeling of urgency is to void and empty your bladder, but this is not so. Urges come and go without emptying your bladder. Remember that they are simply messages, and not commands. You need to think of urgency as a warning only. Then try one of these techniques to help you lessen the urge, which will cause the bladder to relax, and give you more time to get to the bathroom:

- Take some slow, deep breaths through your mouth, concentrating on your breathing; or concentrate on an activity, such as taking a vacation, visiting a friend, enjoying a pleasant memory, counting backwards from 100, or reciting the words of a favorite song or nursery rhyme.
- Tighten or squeeze your pelvic floor muscle quickly several times in a row.

The second bladder training program is "habit training," which is when a person voids whether or not an urge sensation is present. As in the case that follows, habit training can be very successful in persons who do not know when they need to void. *Michael brought his father to his family doctor's office because he couldn't deal with his father's incontinence. His father is 88 years old and suffered a stroke a year ago, but has only a little weakness in his right side. He says he does not know when he has to urinate and Michael finds his father's pants wet with urine several times a day. His father is so embarrassed by the incontinence that he has stopped visiting his friends at the senior center and no longer goes for lunch.*

A caregiver can be invaluable to helping a person keep on a schedule for toileting. Pre-fixed times such as every two hours have been adopted for toileting programs in institutions such as nursing homes. However, a more realistic schedule may be related to certain daily routines such as upon awakening, before or after meals, and at bedtime. If you are caring for a family member who needs to follow a habit training program, here are some tips to promote safe toileting:

- Try to give the person his or her own private bathroom so it is never being used by someone else. If a private bathroom is unavailable or inaccessible, use a bedside commode, urinal, or bedpan.
- Bed height should be sufficient, so that when the person sits on the edge of the bed, feet are flat and the person can easily accomplish going from sitting to standing.
- Keep a clear, direct walking path to the toilet and place night lights along the path.
- Make sure the person can easily use the toilet (e.g., raised toilet seat, grab bars, etc.).
- Make sure the person wears clothing that is easy to remove.
- Locate the bathroom when traveling or carry a portable urinal. Choose seats in restaurants, theaters, etc. that are near a bathroom.
- Use underpads and under-bed sheets on chairs and in the car. Try not to use garbage bags, rubber pads, or shower liners. as these may be too slippery or irritate skin.
- Open windows or use deodorizers to cut down on odors. (A cut-up onion in a room will absorb odors without leaving its own smell, and an open box of baking soda will reduce odors.)

Other Treatments

There are other treatments for incontinence, which are recommended when drugs and behavioral treatments have been unsuccessful. However, these treatments are used only if other treatments have been tried, and may not be indicated in individuals who have other chronic medical problems. They include:

Sling procedures	Surgical method for treating stress UI in men and women involving the placement of a sling, made either of tissue obtained from the person undergoing the sling procedure or of a synthetic mesh or compress.
Percutaneous tibial nerve stimulation (PTNS)	Insertion of a thin needle into the tibial nerve above the ankle to stimulate the nerve by an electrical current. The treatment usually involves weekly visits for 12 weeks and is used in persons with urgency, frequency, and nocturia symptoms.
InterStim or sacral neuromodulation (referred to as a bladder pacemaker)	Treatment for OAB symptoms of urgency and frequency that involves implanting a small battery-driven device. It uses mild electrical pulses (called electrical stimulation) to stimulate the sacral nerves in your lower back, just above the tailbone, that activate or inhibit muscles and organs that contribute to urinary control. This treatment is done in two stages so the success of the treatment on improving symptoms can be tested before actually implanting the device.
Periurethral bulking injections	Involves injecting materials (e.g., Teflon, carbon beads, silicone, a balloon) into the area of the external sphincter to increase compression or closing of the urethra in person with stress incontinence.
Botox injections	Injection of Botox (highly potent neurotoxin) into the dome of the bladder is used to treat persons with OAB symptoms. It has been approved for use in persons who have neurogenic bladder from multiple sclerosis or spinal cord injury.
Artificial urinary sphincter	A mechanical device surgically implanted that consists of a cuff placed around the urethra or bladder neck, a pressure-regulating balloon, and a pump. The device is used to control opening and closing of the urethra manually and is the most commonly used surgical procedure for men with stress incontinence.

Conclusion

Urinary incontinence is the unwanted leakage of urine. Overactive bladder is urinary urgency, usually with frequency and nocturia, with or without urgency incontinence. These bothersome medical conditions affect millions of men and women of all ages. Most suffer the embarrassment in silence, experiencing inconvenience, urine leakage, and the need to frequently access the bathroom. Most do not understand the causes, do not know where to find answers, and believe that there are no solutions. Maybe you are one of these people, hiding your condition from your family, friends, and even from your doctor and other medical providers. If you suffer from UI and/or OAB it is important that you seek help.

Resources

The following groups can be contacted for more information on urinary incontinence.

Alliance for Aging
www.agingresearch.org

Mayo Clinic Resources
www.mayoclinic.com/health/
urinary-incontinence/DS00404/

The Bathroom Diaries
www.thebathroomdiaries.com/

Wellness Partners, LLC
www.seekwellness.com

It's Puzzling...

ALICIA OBERMAN, USA

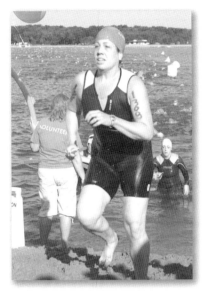

I have thought about writing "my story" countless times. I thought it would be cathartic. I thought it would be inspiring. I thought the words would just flow effortlessly from my fingertips and I wouldn't be able to stop them...

The surprising truth, however, is that I have been staring at a blank screen for hours because I don't even know where to begin. As we all have experienced at one point or another in our lives, there are situations where words fail us. Times when what we feel is so deep, so raw, so exposed, that words are completely inadequate. For me, this is one of those stories.

So, since I am not sure where to start, I gather it is most logical to start at the beginning.

I am a 34-year-old woman who divides her life into two chapters, pre- and post-pelvic reconstructive surgery. The first chapter was my first 33 years, and the second chapter began approximately one year ago. Pre-surgery, after having three 8-pound-plus babies in four and a half years, I suffered from bladder, uterine, and rectal prolapse. I could literally see the bulge of my bladder when I used the bathroom and I could feel my cervix nearly outside of my body. I suffered from stress incontinence, which meant I could not laugh, sneeze, or exert myself in any capacity without leaking urine.

In addition, I could not completely empty my bladder, which meant I had to go to the bathroom at least every hour, if not more often, and to help my bladder along, I had to manually support my bladder with my fingers to empty it further. That and double voiding were the only reasons I wasn't going every 15 minutes. To have a bowel movement I had to rely on stool softeners, and the exact combination of timing of those softeners and a strong cup or two (or sometimes three) of coffee. Finally, sex with my husband was uncomfortable at best and excruciating at worst.

When my youngest daughter was six months old I went to the emergency room twice over the Memorial Day weekend because I could not control the constant overwhelming desire to urinate. The first time they treated me for a bladder infection, even though neither test (the dip nor the culture whose results came later) indicated that I had one. When I went back to the emergency room the second time because there had been no improvement, they were at a loss. Long story short, they decided to insert an indwelling catheter and told me to see my gynecologist for follow-up after the holiday weekend. When I went to my very competent, trusted, and much beloved gynecologist the next day, she too was at a loss. The one thing that was quite clear to her was that I needed to see a urogynecologist as soon as possible. After some trial and error with a pessary at her office, she reinserted the Foley catheter. I used all the favors and clout I could muster to get in to see the recommended urogynecologist the next day.

Without boring you with too many details, the doctor quickly concluded the following: I was experiencing severe bladder spasms brought on by certain physical therapy techniques that I had been doing to "help" my pelvic floor; the Foley catheter needed to come out immediately; I would need a well-fitted pessary to manage my symptoms short-term; and the only mid-term solution would be to have complete pelvic reconstructive surgery. I say "mid-term solution" because as a 32-year-old woman at that time with such a severe prolapse, the likelihood was that the surgery would be effective only so long. In other words, chances are that I will very likely experience prolapse again.

Almost exactly one year after my last child was born, with a five, three, and one-year-old at home, I underwent nearly seven hours of surgery to "fix" me. Without giving you the technical terms, mostly because I cannot pronounce or spell them, I had a hysterectomy, my entire vaginal canal was rebuilt, a mesh sling was inserted to support my urethra to help with my stress incontinence, and a tummy tuck was done. Now some would say the last component was unnecessary, and you could make a valid argument to that effect. However, I was suffering from severe diastasis and also had an umbilical hernia, so in my mind it was in fact essential to complete the reconstruction. It was, however, the one "lollipop" of this entire process; and believe me, given everything else I was going through, it was a psychological must.

After the surgery I faced three grueling months of initial recovery. I had UTI (urinary tract infection) after UTI, I had to self-catheterize for almost three months, and I could not have a bowel movement without maxing out on stool softeners and enemas. I finally had to have a slight revision of the surgery in order to get off the self-cathing. And there was also the pain and exhaustion. The pain was, at times, unbearable. And because the surgery was so long and I lost so much blood, I had to be transfused and was severely anemic for some time after.

Fast-forward one year and here I am. Three months ago, nine months after surgery, I completed my first triathlon. I did so for two reasons. The first is fairly psychologically transparent. An athlete all my life, I needed to prove to myself that I could do it. The second, which is by far the more crucial reason, is that I used it as my own personal marketing campaign to raise awareness and dollars for issues surrounding women's pelvic health and incontinence.

You see, as I recently told a friend who currently suffers from incontinence, albeit for very different reasons, I am extraordinarily frustrated by, and I would go so far as to say angry about, people's overwhelming ignorance when it comes to pelvic health and incontinence. Even in this day and age, when people are often willing to talk about anything and everything, to display details of their lives in any and every public forum, no one wants to talk about this issue. Yet the irony is, once the conversation starts and you get people talking, you can't shut them up.

Simply put, the human body is an extraordinary vessel. Everything has its place and its function. When all is as it should be, it is capable of mind-blowing feats. However, when something is out of place or not working as it should, the consequences can be devastating. Sure, we all suffer through aches and pains, and sometimes feel a bit out of sorts; but there is nothing more basic than having control of your bladder and bowels. When there is a kink in that function, or that system breaks, the physical and, more importantly, the psychological consequences can be devastating.

For those of you reading this who do not have issues with eliminating, the next time you feel the urge to go, please stop and imagine what it would be like if you could not just sit down on a toilet, do your business, wash your hands, and go back to your life.

Imagine you can't just go to a restaurant, have a couple of glasses of wine with friends, eat whatever you feel like eating on the menu, go home, and be intimate with your spouse any way and as many times as you would like, and then let all of that run its natural course through your system. If I allow myself an evening like that, here is what runs through my mind, even after surgery and recovery: "OK, if I have the glasses of wine that is fine, but it will irritate my bladder so I have to make sure I have enough water to compensate and dilute that wine. But if I have too much water, I am going to have to go to the bathroom all night. And I have to be careful during all of these calculations to not let my bladder get too full because I have a more difficult time emptying my bladder when it is full, and there is more pressure on my urethra. Also, I can't eat anything too spicy or acidic because this too will irritate my bladder, so I have to decide which is more important, the wine or the food? Finally, I can go home and have sex with my husband after this rare night out, but if I have too much sex, or it is in the wrong position, I risk having bladder spasms that feel fairly similar to a UTI without the burning. If I overdo it with the sex, it will take me about three or four days of bladder training to get the resulting bladder spasms under control. And finally, through all of this, I need to make sure I eat enough fiber and drink just enough coffee and water to keep my bowels moving without the aid of stool softeners. And yes, let's remember here, I am 34 years old and will have to think about this the rest of my life."

So, that takes us to the question that people ask me most often, which is "So, are you finally a hundred percent?" I have come to realize that I am not sure that any one of us is one hundred percent ever, if we are truly engaged in our lives and honest with ourselves. But that existential analysis aside, if they are only asking about my pelvic issues, as you can see, I will never again function the same way I functioned before I had children. It is not something I spend all day every day thinking about, but I will always live my life with a heightened sense of awareness of giving my body the tools to work at its highest capacity. I constantly have to be conscious of what goes in, what goes out, how I move, and most importantly, not forgetting to breathe.

And despite all of this, I feel tremendously fortunate. I can leave my house, go to work, be with my family and friends, and no one would be the wiser of my experiences if I didn't want to share them. But as anyone who has spent time with me in the last year knows, not a single day goes by that I do not try to be a voice for those who do not feel comfortable speaking for themselves. If you do not think that incontinence is a prevalent issue in this country, just go to your local drugstore and look through the aisle that displays products to deal with incontinence. It is huge. And, despite the stereotype and public perception, it is not just older people looking at those products. You will see all types of people: men, women, young, old, able-bodied and disabled, and needless to say, all races and demographics. And while incontinence is not literally life threatening, which is often a response that I get when I lend my voice to the issue, I would remind you, as a friend reminded me, that there are other types of death that may in fact be worse than the actual thing.

Another question I get often is whether I am angry that I have had to go through all of this. My answer is quite the opposite. The easy answer to that question is that there are many, many people in this world who are suffering far worse than this. But the more important and complicated answer is that I feel extraordinarily lucky. I have been given a gift. I am young, I am articulate, I am unabashedly candid, and I have access to resources, intellectually, personally and professionally, to dramatically change the conversation surrounding pelvic health and incontinence. I had this experience so that I can shift the paradigm. To look at it any other way to me is simply impossible.

I have three little girls, all with pelvic floors and all with my genes. When they are my age, or when they are older, if they encounter pelvic floor or incontinence issues, whether "fixable" or not, they have to live in a world where they do not feel stigmatized, inadequate, or ashamed. As a mother, the alternative is not an option.

CHAPTER 4

Bowel Control and Managing a Misbehaving Bowel

CHRISTINE NORTON, PhD, RN

EDITOR'S NOTE: This chapter is for you if you have difficulty controlling your bowels. You may have urgency (needing to rush to find a toilet), or have "accidents" when you don't make it there in time. Or you may find that you leak from the bowel without realising it, or pass flatus (gas/wind) without meaning to. Or you may not feel secure in your bowel control, even though you never actually leak.

You will probably have already tried many of the ideas in this chapter, and we presume that you have had some professional health care for your bowel. This chapter is to help you re-visit some ideas and alert you to others that you may not have come across before. Understanding what may have gone wrong is often the first step in coming to terms with and tackling a problem.

All of us are born without control of our bowels. Children usually learn bowel control before they are five years of age, but this varies a lot. Most adults are able to take bowel control for granted and need to give it little thought except for the few minutes a day that are spent emptying the bowel. However, bowel control is actually a complex and not completely understood process, involving delicate coordination of many different nerves and muscles.

Our gut breaks down (digests) the food that we eat to extract nutrients, which are then absorbed. Any parts of food that the body cannot use are processed, water is removed, and the waste is expelled as faeces ("stools").

This process starts at the mouth and finishes at the anus or back passage (Figure 1). Food is broken down by chewing. It is then swallowed, passes down the gullet (oesophagus), and reaches the stomach. The small bowel, or small intestines, is the part of the bowel where the useful parts of food are absorbed in the blood stream and taken to where they are needed.

Figure 1. The digestive system

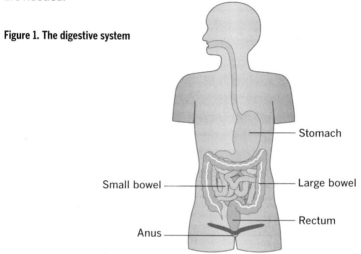

Stomach

Small bowel

Large bowel

Rectum

Anus

The small bowel delivers one to two pints (500-1,000 ml) of waste to the colon per day. The colon or large bowel is the waste processing part of the system (Figure 2). This waste is the consistency of thick soup when it enters the beginning of the colon. It is the job of the colon to absorb fluid from this waste and, as it moves around the colon, to gradually form it into stools (also called faeces or bowel movements). Stool consistency can vary between hard lumps to very soft or mushy. The consistency often depends on how long the stools have been in the colon and how much water has been absorbed from them. Ideally stools should be formed into soft smooth sausage-shapes which are comfortable to pass.

Figure 2. The large bowel

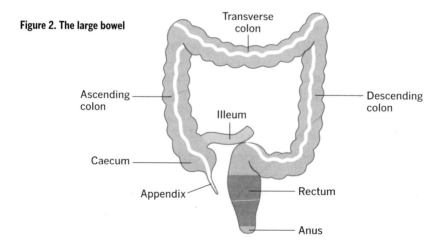

Transverse colon

Ascending colon

Descending colon

Illeum

Caecum

Appendix

Rectum

Anus

Figure 3. Mass movements in the colon

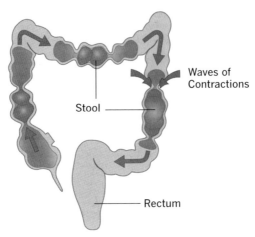

Waves of
Contractions

Stool

Rectum

The left side of the colon and the rectum are the "storage tank" at the end of the large bowel. Normally the rectum is relatively empty. Stool does not enter the rectum from the colon on a continuous basis, but as a result of mass movements, which happen from time to time, especially before the need to go to the toilet is experienced. These mass movements are major waves of pressure, which can move stool through the whole length of the colon, like toothpaste being squeezed along a tube (Figure 3). Often a large part of the contents of the colon arrives in the rectum at once. The lining of the bowel produces fluid called mucus (a bit like the saliva in your mouth) which lubricates the movement of stools along the colon.

These mass movements are often triggered by the so-called "gastro-colic response." Food arriving in the stomach when you eat a meal sets off a pressure wave in the colon some minutes later. This can lead to the need to empty the bowel, sometimes urgently, soon after eating. For many people the bowel is relatively quiet at night. The first meal of the day, together with the physical activity involved in getting out of bed and washing and dressing, stimulates contractions in the colon and mass movements. This leads to a "call to stool," the feeling that the bowel needs emptying, shortly after breakfast.

Food usually takes an average of one to three days to be processed between the mouth and the anus. Up to 90% of that time is spent in the colon.

How Often Should I Empty the Bowel?

There is no right or wrong answer to this. There is a very wide range of "normal" bowel function between different people. It is by no means essential to have one bowel movement per day, and indeed it is probably a minority of the total population who has this. Some people always go several times per day; others have several days between bowel actions.

Perception of what is normal is based on personal experiences and growing up with other people. Most of us do not discuss our bowel habits with our friends, or even our family. A few people become obsessed with the need for a daily bowel action and spend excessive amounts of time in the toilet or take laxatives to achieve this. Often this is unnecessary.

Normal Bowel Emptying

When stool enters the rectum the internal anal sphincter muscle automatically relaxes and opens up the top of the anal canal. This is normal and allows stool to enter the upper anal canal to be "sampled" by the very sensitive nerve cells in the upper anal canal (Figure 4). People with normal sensation can easily tell the difference between wind (gas, also called *flatus*), which can safely be passed if it is socially convenient without fear of soiling, diarrhoea (very loose or runny stools needing urgent attention and access to a toilet), and a normal stool. Most people just know what is in the rectum without really having to think about it.

Figure 4. Internal sphincter relaxes when the rectum is full

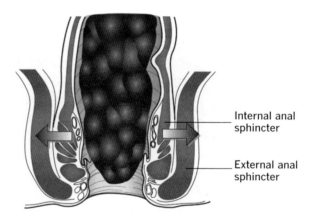

Internal anal
sphincter

External anal
sphincter

Around the internal anal sphincter is the *external anal sphincter,* which is much thicker. This is the muscle around the anus that you can deliberately squeeze. Just like the muscles in the arm or leg, a person can decide when to use this muscle.

If a normal stool is sensed and it is not convenient to find a toilet at that moment, bowel emptying is delayed by squeezing the external anal sphincter. Squeezing the external sphincter ensures that the stool is not simply expelled as soon as it enters the rectum, and in fact the stool is pushed back up out of the anal canal (Figure 5). For most people this is not a deliberate action – you should not need to think, "I must squeeze my anal sphincter muscles so that I do not have a bowel accident" – but this is actually what you do, subconsciously without really thinking about it.

Figure 5. External sphincter muscle contraction

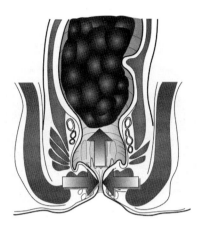

This external sphincter squeeze does not need to last all the time until the toilet is found. Stool is pushed back into the rectum, and the rectum relaxes so that the urge to empty the bowel is resisted and wears off.

For most people, an urge to empty the bowel is felt, but if the time and place are not right, it is possible for them to delay bowel emptying, and the feeling of needing to go wears off very soon. Most people can then forget about the bowel for a while, and some can put off bowel emptying almost indefinitely, but may get reminders that the bowel is full at intervals until it is emptied. Continually resisting the urge to empty the bowel or ignoring the call to stool can lead to constipation, as the longer the stools stay in the colon and rectum, the more fluid is absorbed and the harder the stools will become.

Causes of Bowel Control Difficulties

The system described above is delicately balanced, depending on long nerve pathways and muscles all working together. Unfortunately, there are many things that can go wrong with it to either hinder development of control or lessen control once it has developed. The most common problems are:

Damage to the Nerves

Nerves control both the feelings (sensations) from the bowel and the ability to do something about a full rectum (such as squeezing the external sphincter). Nerves can be damaged from birth, or later in life.

Damage to the Muscles

As described above, muscle control is crucial to bowel control. The muscles of the anus can be damaged by childbirth, surgery, or an accident.

An "Overactive" Bowel or Loose Stools

Some people have a bowel that is a lot more active than other peoples', or is sensitive and easily upset (maybe by certain foods or stress). Others have bowel conditions like colitis that cause diarrhoea. If stools are loose, or the activity in the bowel is causing the rectum to fill much more often, this will be more difficult to control.

Severe Constipation

If the lower bowel becomes overloaded with hard stools, this irritates the bowel lining, which then produces more mucus. If the rectum is full continuously, the muscles of the anus relax and the liquid mucus can leak out. This can be mistaken for diarrhoea.

Managing a Misbehaving Bowel

There are no simple solutions to the difficult problem of an unpredictable or leaking bowel. This book is written primarily for people who have tried everything and still have a problem. However, it is worth reviewing whether you really have tried everything, and sometimes it is worth re-visiting options that you have tried and discarded. This chapter outlines options that people have found helpful. More details can be found from the sources found in the Appendix at the end of the book, Worldwide Resources.

Getting Into a Predictable Routine

Most people find that their bowel goes to sleep at night and wakes up when they wake up in the morning. The bowel is stimulated by movement and eating or drinking and for most people mass movements are most likely after their first meal of the day. If you are on your way to work when this happens, this can spell disaster.

You can capitalise on this increased activity in the morning by attempting to "train" your bowel to empty at a predictable time when you are near a toilet. It is important NOT to skip breakfast. Eating and drinking will activate your bowel so that you can empty it. It really does not matter what you eat, but eat something with a couple of hot or cold drinks. You will need to be near a toilet after breakfast, which may mean getting up a bit earlier than usual if you normally get up and go straight out of the house.

About twenty to thirty minutes after breakfast (sooner if you feel the urge), sit on the toilet and try to empty the bowel. Do this, not by holding your breath and straining, but by using the muscles in your abdomen (Figure 6). Locate these muscles by putting your hands on your waist and coughing – you should feel the muscles of your waist bulging out. Now deliberately "make your waist wide" by bulging these muscles outwards and gently, but firmly, push downwards and backwards. At the same time deliberately relax the muscles around the anus. Keep pushing without holding your breath. Don't spend more than about five minutes on the toilet.

Figure 6. Emptying the bowel

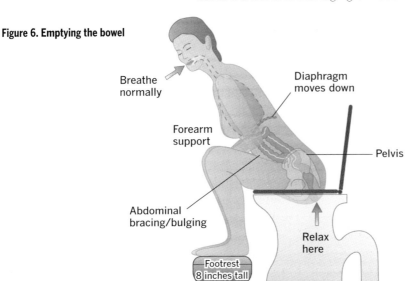

Breathe normally

Diaphragm moves down

Forearm support

Pelvis

Abdominal bracing/bulging

Relax here

Footrest 8 inches tall

If at first nothing happens, don't give up! Try this every day for at least a week. If you are still getting no results, consider stimulating the bowel into acting at a convenient time (see section on Taking Control, page 63).

Bowel Retraining

For people with frequency and urgency (needing to rush to the toilet), it can help to practice holding on and waiting once you feel the urge. This can feel very difficult, if not impossible, at first. So to make it easier you can start the retraining sitting on the toilet. When you feel that urgent need, get onto the toilet and then WAIT before letting go. Squeeze the anal muscles (see pelvic floor exercises in the following section) and hold on as long as you can. You may be surprised how long you can actually wait.

Even if this is only a few seconds to start with, keep trying and holding. Once you can reliably hold for a minute, start to delay sitting down. Gradually get further and further away from the toilet while you are holding on. The idea is to overcome those feelings of panic when you feel the urgency. Once you know that you can hold, the anxiety feels less and the urgency improves. This can take weeks or even months to achieve, so you have to be persistent and not give up too soon. It is best to practice this when you are at home or somewhere else safe, as it will undermine your confidence if you have an accident while you are trying to hold on. You might like to use a low dose of medication such as loperamide to help you with this (see page 64).

Pelvic Floor Exercises

These exercises are designed to strengthen the muscles around the anus. It is important to learn to do the exercises in the right way, and to check from time to time that you are still doing them correctly (See Box 1 on page 63).

Sit comfortably with your knees slightly apart. Now imagine that you are trying to stop yourself passing wind from the bowel. To do this you must squeeze the muscle around the back passage. Try squeezing and lifting that muscle as tightly as you can, as if you are really worried that you are about to leak. You should be able to feel the muscle move. Your buttocks, abdomen, and legs should not move much at all. You should be aware of the skin around the back passage tightening and being pulled up and away from your chair. Really try to feel this. You are now exercising your anal sphincter muscles. You should not need to hold your breath when you tighten the muscles!

When you squeeze as tightly as you can, you cannot hold it there for very long, and it will not get you safely to the toilet because the anal sphincter muscle will get tired very quickly. So now squeeze more gently (try to imagine squeezing half-way to the maximum). Feel how much longer you can hold it than at the maximum squeeze. You can hold a squeeze at half-way longer than you can hold a squeeze at maximum.

Sometimes you may need to activate the muscles very quickly (for example if you are going to pass wind). To help with this, do some "fast-twitch" exercises – squeeze and relax as quickly as you can.

At first it is probably a good idea to set aside some time for these exercises and really concentrate on getting them right. But quite soon they should become easy to do wherever you are. Nobody need know what you are doing! As your muscles strengthen, you should be able to hold each squeeze for longer and do more repeats. Muscles get stronger by exercising them often and hard (just like going to the gym – if you do what is easy you do not improve). So the amount of exercise needs to be individualized; gradually doing a little more and feeling that you have worked hard should be your objective.

Try to get into the habit of doing your exercises with things you do regularly: every time you touch water if you are at home, every time you answer the phone if you are at the office – something you do often. If you are unsure that you are exercising the right muscle, put a finger on the anus as you squeeze to check. You should feel a gentle lift and squeeze if you are exercising the right muscle. Or look at the area in a mirror – you should see the anus pucker up as you squeeze it.

Use your muscles when you need them – pull up the muscles if you feel urgency and that you are about to leak. But remember that you cannot hold your tightest squeeze for very long, so you are better to use a gentler squeeze that you can hold for longer. Your control will gradually improve. Once you have regained control of your bowel, don't forget your exercises. Continue to do them a few times each day to ensure that the problem does not come back.

Remember, you can do these exercises wherever you are – nobody need know what you are doing!

Box 1: Practising Your Pelvic Floor Exercises

1. Sit, stand, or lie with your knees slightly apart. Slowly tighten and pull up the anal muscles as tightly as you can. Hold tightened for at least five seconds, and then relax for at least ten seconds.

   Repeat at least five times. This will work on the **strength** of your muscles.

2. Next, pull the muscles up to about half of their maximum squeeze. See how long you can hold this. Then relax for at least ten seconds.

   Repeat at least five times. This will work on the **endurance** or staying power of your muscles.

3. Pull up the muscles as quickly and tightly as you can and then relax and pull up again, and see how many times you can do this before you get tired. Try for at least five quick pull-ups.

4. Do all of these exercises – five as hard as you can, five as long as you can, and as many quick pull-ups as you can – at least three times every day.

5. As the muscles get stronger, you will find that you can hold for longer than five seconds, and that you can do more pull-ups each time without the muscle getting tired.

6. It takes time for exercise to make muscles stronger. You may need to exercise regularly for several months before the muscles gain their full strength.

Biofeedback and Electrical Stimulation

If the anal muscles are very weak, it can be difficult to achieve very much with exercises on your own. Your health professional may suggest using computer equipment to help you locate and exercise your muscles (biofeedback). This equipment usually involves a small probe to measure your muscle pressure and a screen to give you feedback to tell you if you are using the right muscles or not. Sometimes electrical stimulation – using a small probe and a very low and safe electrical current from a battery to help you feel and exercise the muscles – may also be suggested.

Taking Control by Choosing When Your Bowel Will Empty

All of the following options should only be used on the advice of your health care practitioner.

Suppositories and Enemas. Suppositories are small, soft, and bullet-shaped. They can be inserted into the rectum using a finger. Some are simple lubricants; others contain a mild irritant medication. Enemas can be very small (5 ml) or larger volumes (100 ml+) of water or medicated liquid in a squeezable bottle with a nozzle to insert into the rectum. The aim of both suppositories and enemas is to start the rectum emptying at a time convenient for you. It is usual to insert suppositories or an enema lying on your side, or sitting on the toilet. With a bit of practice you may find that the timing for emptying of the bowel that results is very predictable, thus enabling you to plan your day more easily.

Laxatives. There are literally dozens of different laxatives that you can take by mouth to help if you are constipated or have hard stools. Some act as stool softeners; others stimulate the muscles of the bowel wall to push stool along more effectively. This may help you to have a predictable bowel action. However, many people find that laxatives taken by mouth are a bit unpredictable and can leave you waiting near a toilet all day if your control is not good. Laxatives should not be taken on a regular basis without medical advice.

Anti-diarrhoea Medication. People with bowel incontinence who also have loose stool or diarrhoea often find that taking medication to firm up the stools is helpful and may decrease urgency and bowel incontinence. The most commonly used medication is loperamide, which can be used on a regular basis if needed, or can also be taken just for specific activities such as a journey or eating out. If you think that this may be helpful, you should discuss this with your doctor.

Irrigation. Specially designed kits for washing out the lower bowel with one to two pints of regular tap water are being developed. It is not yet clear exactly which bowel problems will respond well to bowel irrigation.

Manual Evacuation. Many people with neurological conditions such as a low spinal cord injury or spina bifida find that the rectum simply does not empty on its own and they need to use a finger to help stool out. Doing this gently on a regular basis (every one to two days) with a gloved, lubricated finger keeps the rectum empty and therefore incontinence becomes much less likely.

Managing Gas

Controlling gas is often the most difficult aspect of bowel control. Much of the advice above applies to controlling gas as much as controlling stool. The exercises and routine outlined above have been found helpful. Many people find that diet has a big influence on how much gas your bowel produces and how it smells. Gassy foods vary between individuals, so it is worth experimenting yourself. But it will be impossible to eliminate gas altogether. The "fast-twitch" pelvic floor exercises may help to speed up your reaction time if you feel gas coming, but many people do not have sufficient sensation to feel gas.

It is worth mentioning that you will be a lot more aware of your body functions than people who are around you. Most people pass gas ten to twenty times each day, yet how often do you notice anyone else doing this? In reality, most people are tied up in their own lives and activities and thoughts and are unlikely to notice your accidental passing of gas.

Surgery to Improve Bowel Control

There are several operations that help with bowel control in some circumstances. By the time you are reading this book, we assume that you have explored all possible options with you healthcare providers and have decided that none of these is right for you, or you do not want to go down the surgical route, or you have tried surgery and it has not worked for you. However, there may be some operations you have not yet considered. Options include:

> Sphincter repair
> Sacral nerve stimulation
> Artificial bowel sphincter
> Stimulated gracioplasty
> Ostomy formation

We do not go into more detail here, but if you are interested to find out more, try the IFFGD website (for details, see appendix Worldwide Resources).

Tips on Food and Drinks

It may be helpful to keep a food and bowel diary for about a week to see if you can spot any patterns. Food generally takes one to three days to pass through your system, so if you have a bad day it may be what you ate yesterday that has upset you, not today's meal. As eating and drinking stimulates the bowel to work, it may be worth adjusting your eating pattern to make sure you can access a toilet after meals. But try not to become obsessed with what and when you eat as this can lead to imbalances in your diet.

What Might Help

This is very individual. Research has suggested that some people with poor bowel control do better with a diet low in fibre; others have fewer symptoms with a high fibre diet. It is certainly worth experimenting if you have not done so already. If you have irritable bowel syndrome, with bouts of diarrhoea, you may find diet can regulate your symptoms (see the IFFGD website in the appendix Worldwide Resources).

What Might Make Things Worse

Caffeine (in coffee, tea, cola, and chocolate) is a gut stimulant and may make urgency or loose stool worse. Fibre is a problem for some people but not others. Spicy foods, onions, green vegetables, salads, citrus, and many other things are sometimes to blame.

Watch Your Weight

There is some scientific evidence that heavier people are more prone to bowel incontinence. Extra weight can put extra strain on your muscles and extra pressure on your bowel. Of course it is easier said than done to lose weight, so do think about getting some professional help if you are struggling with your weight. For some people losing weight can really help with both bowel and bladder control.

Hope For the Future

It can be very difficult to live with an unpredictable or leaking bowel and there are few perfect solutions. However, new options are being actively developed, including medications, surgery, and products, so it is worth checking from time to time to see if anything new has been introduced.

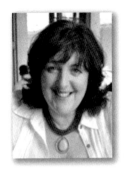

Living with Faecal Incontinence

LOUISE MOTT, UK

I was happily married and a busy graduate midwife when I had my first child in 1997. I had spent the previous years working as a midwife in a busy hospital. Most women in the UK have their babies with a midwife in the hospital, or occasionally at home. I had managed and delivered over 120 babies myself. I was used to dealing with the less glamorous side of childbirth such as perineal tears, and was proficient at suturing them. I had also rotated onto the postnatal area where we cared for women and their babies following birth. I loved my job and planned to return within a year after giving birth.

I had a difficult and protracted labour that resulted in a forceps delivery of a healthy baby boy. I was told I had a second-degree tear. However, the next few days in hospital were excruciating; even walking was difficult. I was surprised that the women I had cared for could cope with such pain. It was in those first few days that I had my first episode of incontinence. There was no warning. I was horrified and really embarrassed. I felt dirty and unattractive, and so I didn't tell anyone.

My incontinence continued after I went home, but trying to manage a new baby was enough and therefore I kept putting the incontinence to the back of my mind, even though I was cleaning myself up more and more often. I still had a lot of pain as well. I didn't go out at all and asked my husband to do the grocery shopping – I told him my reclusive behaviour was because I was struggling with the baby.

When my doctor saw me at six weeks for a postnatal check she inquired if I had resumed sex. I said no I hadn't because of the pain and the incontinence. She told me it was still early and not to worry. I felt awkward for bringing it up and also invalidated. I decided right then and there to keep it to myself in the future. As a qualified nurse and midwife I know better; but incontinence is an extremely taboo subject. In addition, I was in denial about how bad it was getting.

After six months my incontinence was almost daily, causing me to feel dirty and unattractive. I was paranoid that I smelled bad, hence sex was out of the question and the fear of "accidents" made me reclusive. One day

I had just had a major incontinent episode when my husband came home unexpectedly and found me crying. I lied by telling him something on the TV had upset me. He knew I didn't usually watch daytime TV and said there had to be something else going on. I broke down and told him everything, fully expecting him to recoil in horror and disgust. He did the opposite – he looked relieved and hugged me. He had been afraid, imagining what could be wrong. Now he felt included and empowered to offer help. That very night he held my hand when we went to see the doctor.

That doctor's visit resulted in consultations with gynaecologists, surgeons, and biomedical testing on my bowel and bottom at St. Mark's Hospital in London. A scan revealed an undiagnosed and unrepaired fourth degree tear. The experts at St. Mark's recommended biofeedback, but my surgeon didn't agree. Sadly, because I was depressed, didn't have enough information, and lacked a well-informed advocate, I went along with the surgeon's advice. I just wanted it to go away, so I elected to have an anal sphincter repair.

Given my nursing background, I knew I needed antibiotics before this surgery, but the surgeon said it was not necessary. Three days post-op I got a terrible infection, causing the repair to burst open and leave a gaping wound. Due to the infection, more surgery was not possible. It took four and a half months to heal. My incontinence was terrible and caused the wound to break down often. My depression got much worse.

It was now nearly two years after giving birth and I still had not resumed sexual relations. When I asked for a second opinion I was referred back to St. Mark's. There I met two people who changed my life: a colorectal surgeon who vowed to work with me until I had a marked improvement, and a nurse continence specialist who talked frankly, wanted to help, and was proactive – the advocate I needed.

I completed biofeedback training and tried several medications, anal plugs, incontinence pads, never-ending Kegel exercises, bowel wash-outs, and enemas – all to no avail. A colostomy or sacral nerve stimulation were not options because I have a blood clotting disorder, discovered during my anal sphincter repair, making further interventions unsafe.

Whilst receiving biofeedback I joined a self-help group for women with bowel incontinence. I found it very helpful to talk with people experiencing the same problems, to listen to the coping strategies of others – I felt a sense of belonging. However, I had still not resumed sexual relations (some feelings are hard to overcome) and my long-suffering husband was showing signs of despair. I called Relate, the marriage guidance counsellors in England, and they offered us a psychosexual therapist. After a lot of upset, false starts, and fear, we managed to commence tentative and then full relations. The unexpected, but very happy result of this was that I became pregnant again. It had taken over four years for me to resume a normal sexual relationship because of a stigma that meant I couldn't talk about my problem.

Another life changing event occurred when the self-help group leader asked me to speak to nurses at a local university for their mental health study day. The subject was "quality of life issues in women with faecal incontinence." I was a relative recluse who had not been able to work and, because of depression and absolute fear of being incontinent, had not been very social for years. With the self-help group leader's unwavering support, my extremely understanding and supportive husband's encouragement, and a lot of Imodium, I stood in front of twenty people and told my story. I was extremely nervous and this made my bowel very irritable; I went to the toilet about ten times before I started, but I DID IT.

That one thirty-minute talk enabled me to see that I could do something useful. It totally empowered me, and I truly felt I could offer a valid perspective that would have a positive impact on other sufferers. When asked to do more talks I decided to put my midwifery background to work, and changed the format of my presentations to involve helping midwives and nurses detect women who were suffering in silence, whether in hospital or in the community. Since then I have spoken many times at several universities about incontinence, and have presented my story on video as part of a "Foundations of Gastrointestinal Nursing" degree course.

I now live with my family in Vancouver, Canada. This move presented me with a new dilemma; did I tell my "secret" to my new friends, or did I live hoping not to be exposed? That is still a difficult choice for me because everyone reacts differently to the information, and dealing with their responses sometimes takes a lot of inner strength. I am still incontinent on a regular basis, but now try to live my life to the fullest. I am still concerned with "smells" and am more reserved in the bedroom, but a willing participant. I went camping this year with my family for the first time since I was a child – something I thought I would never do again. I loved it.

If I have an accident in public I have learned to stay calm, and as soon as possible get to a restroom to deal with the situation. I decided I would rule my life and not let incontinence rule me. It took a lot of adjustments and time to get here, but now I am my own advocate and trust my own judgements.

CHAPTER 5

How We View Our Own Bodies

RONALD H. ROZENSKY, PhD, STEVEN M. TOVIAN, PhD, PAMELA DUBYAK, MS

EDITOR'S NOTE: Many people with incontinence struggle with more than just the physical symptoms: they also struggle with self-confidence. Low self-confidence can lead to feelings of hopelessness and a perceived loss of power. This chapter examines how incontinence can affect our body image, and provides strategies for accepting how your body functions and improving your body image.

The media and the advertising industry bombard us daily with pictures of beautiful, perfect people who are engaging in fun-filled activities. It is unlikely that these models are considered to be anything but that, models to emulate; that is, able-bodied individuals without day-to-day problems to manage. It is doubtful that when we look at these images, we consider these people as having any limitations on their activities. This would surely include little thought that an active, involved person might have to manage problems with continence.

We learn as children that "having accidents" and "wetting our pants" is unacceptable. If this happens as an adult, many people believe that they must have done something wrong. It is possible that you might see yourself or your body as "dirty" or "wrong" because you cannot control your bladder. Over the course of this chapter, we will offer you some ideas on how to challenge these thoughts and how to modify them to be more positive about your body image, your self-esteem, and yourself.

Body Image

Body image is related to how we see ourselves (who is that person in the mirror and how does he or she look?). Body image has been described as the mental image or "picture" an individual has of his or her own body. This image includes our thoughts and feelings about our outward appearance as well as how we think about our internal organs and our body's workings. Additionally, our reactions to our physical anatomy and our bodily processes are also part of our body image. These reactions can be related to experiences such as "growth spurts" in our height as a child or adolescent, fluctuations in our weight throughout our life, the first time a young boy notices facial hair or a young woman begins to develop breasts. And our body image is related to how we react to how we *think* others see us.

A positive sense of "self" depends on many things. How we manage any difficulties we encounter has a great impact on how we feel about ourselves. If we have a distortion in our body image, that distortion can impact how we feel about ourselves and in turn can impact our willingness to interact with others.

Body image is very important to how we relate to other people. Our image of our body changes over time due to new experiences. Issues differ across the different stages of our lifespan; what is important to a teenager looking in the mirror or wondering about a group of friends looking back at him or her is very different from what is important to an older adult focused on the normal aging process or managing an acute or ongoing illness.

People who feel confident about how they look may feel more confident interacting with other people and this, in turn, can impact how we develop interpersonal relationships. On the other hand, people who feel uncertain about themselves may be less likely to interact comfortably with others because they are afraid of being rejected or hurt emotionally. Body image can play an important role in how we think, how we feel about ourselves, and how we interact with other people. The social and cultural context in which we live helps dictate how we see ourselves. Also, how we interpret ourselves within that social context impacts how we feel and what we are willing do to socially. For example, 17th century artist Peter Paul Rubens painted portraits of full-figured, "Rubenesque" women, considered back then as alluring and attractive. Today, as we see in the media, our culture values thinner women as attractive, not those who are Rubenesque. This is an example of how cultural *interpretation* can dictate how we feel about our own bodies. Managing one's reaction to perceived cultural norms and how those norms might impact how we see ourselves is something we can control. It is *our* interpretation – that is, how we think and feel – that we can use to moderate how we feel about ourselves.

Incontinence and Body Image

Incontinence can alter your perception of your body image. Even if no one directly knows you must manage the challenges of incontinence on a daily basis, you might interpret your incontinence as having an impact on your body image and thus feel uncomfortable with yourself, especially around others. You might feel that you appear "different" to others because your bodily processes are not "behaving" as you might wish (e.g., "I cannot control my bladder; something is wrong with *me* and everyone will know.") This is your *interpretation* of the situation. Imagine how different you might feel if you were to say to yourself, "I have developed incontinence due to having (fill in the reason). This is a difficult situation to manage at times, but I am proud of how I have faced it and I have to keep on with my activities to enjoy my life." Imagine how you would feel about yourself and your image of yourself if you said that! Even if someone says directly to you something you feel uncomfortable about, how you react and how you feel about what they have said are equally within *your* control based upon how you interpret their remarks.

In order to have a positive body image when you must manage incontinence, you need to restructure your body image and self-perceptions to integrate physical changes you may be experiencing in a manner that does not impact you negatively. By accepting these changes to how your body works, you will reduce any feelings of sadness, anxiety, anger, and social withdrawal. "Accepting" does *not* mean you have to like or endorse these changes. Accepting means acknowledging that you have something that you must manage so that you can minimize its impact on your activities, comfort, and self-image. Managing how you think and feel about your body and yourself can be learned and put into practice in a way to minimize the negative impact on your feelings about yourself and your day-to-day quality of life.

Body Image and the Personal Response

Although incontinence affects each individual person in a unique way, many people with incontinence report many similar feelings. For example, many people with incontinence report feeling isolated, depressed, and anxious, and put a lot of energy into trying to appear as "normal" as possible by doing things that either limit causes of urinating (fluid restrictions) or avoiding social situations so as to not "let on" that they must visit the restroom often. Some people with incontinence are not able to see their incontinence as a medical problem only, but feel that there is something "wrong" with them because they cannot control their bladder or bowel and therefore feel guilty about this. Other people with incontinence view their condition as a symbol of their lack of moral worth and link incontinence with personal failings (e.g., being overweight). These feelings can have a large impact on an individual's ability to manage his or her incontinence. Loss of control over one's body, after being taught as a child that having accidents is "bad," can result in a person questioning his or her personal identity and feeling anxious and ashamed. While you might be thinking that some of these thoughts are extreme and untrue, for many people actually recognizing these thoughts as extreme during a given moment of stress is challenging. It can be difficult to focus on the nature of these thoughts and challenge the thoughts and their impact on our feelings and actions, but it is possible to establish new ways of managing our thoughts.

Body Image and the Sexual Response

Body image and sexual response are interrelated. Each day we see images of sexual myths in the media: only beautiful, healthy people are sexually active; people with disabilities are absent from these TV and advertising images. It is understandable that incontinence can interfere with the sexual response and how you see your body. For example, a person with incontinence may need to visit the bathroom prior to or during sexual relations. They may need to discuss "leaking" with their partner in order to explain what can happen and why. Incontinence may even make a person question his or her sexual desirability and sexual abilities. Simply avoiding thinking about these issues may add to the problem and, without open discussion with a partner, you might conclude that your body is less attractive. For example, if you feel uncomfortable due to your incontinence and you then choose to avoid sexual intimacy, do you then conclude that your body is unattractive? "Oh, we don't have sex anymore; it must be because I have become unattractive." What if you discussed incontinence and sexuality with your partner and he or she said, "Oh, well, I wish you didn't leak, but I still find you sexy. I wondered why you were avoiding *me*!" If you don't ask, you will have no chance to challenge your negative body image.

> " *Self-pity gets you nowhere. One must have the adventurous daring to accept oneself as a bundle of possibilities and undertake the most interesting game in the world making the most of one's best.* "
>
> —Harry Emerson Fosdick

Body Image and the Social Response

Some people with incontinence report challenges with maintaining friendships. For example, the fear of the presence of odors or sights (e.g., change of clothes and personal hygiene items) can disrupt close relationships when friends or loved ones do not understand. Some people report that friends they have told about their incontinence have reacted negatively. Many people with incontinence will arrange their schedules in order to avoid spending time with other people (e.g., to avoid the possibility of leakage in front of others). Some may feel isolated and alone, because they feel that others may not respond positively and/or that they will not be able to control their symptoms. Isolation and the resulting decrease in rewarding experiences can result in increased symptoms of depression and limit the possibility of positive experiences.

Having a negative body image can also impair your ability to function within the workplace. Many people who experience incontinence do not feel comfortable telling their colleagues about their condition because they are concerned that they will be viewed poorly. Sometimes people assume that everyone has a negative image of them because they, themselves, have a negative image of their own body. They may be hyperaware of accidents and odor at work because they are concerned that these symptoms will affect their job status or the possibility of promotion.

Do you think that people at work actually know of your incontinence? Do you know that they view this as negative? How do you know that your boss is not incontinent? Did her incontinence interfere with her "moving up the ladder" at work? Your boss may have a spouse or parent who has to manage incontinence, and may well be very supportive of your situation. You can challenge yourself in these situations to make certain that you are not making assumptions about others because you, yourself, are uncomfortable with your body and the need to manage both your incontinence and your reactions to it. Try telling yourself: "My quality of work is not less because I am incontinent. I work hard and my place at work is based on my skills, not my bodily functions."

Managing Body Image and Incontinence

How can one manage body image issues and incontinence? *Coping* is a term often used when talking about managing one's reactions to illness, disability, crisis, or even natural disasters like floods and severe storms. Coping describes what you do about a problem to become calm, establish emotional balance, or return to the feelings that were present before the problem began. This has three important parts. First, there is a recognized problem from which one seeks relief. Second, there is what one does or does not do about the problem. Third, there is a result or outcome, which may or may not be effective in actually managing one's reaction to the problem or situation.

Coping may be seen as your action or behavior, as your way to manage, master, tolerate, reduce, or minimize demands or stress coming from the outside world or even from within yourself – responses that tax, drain, or challenge your resources. Coping is a series of related steps or strategies and not a single set of independent actions. Coping does not mean merely feeling better or less troubled by a problem. It is also important to know what you did to solve the problem. This fosters a sense of increased control and self-management.

Coping is something we routinely do every day. We hardly notice it unless a problem continues and we start to feel increased emotional distress. Look for some unresolved problem whenever emotional distress occurs. For example, try to remember an occasion recently when you felt shame, humiliation, depression, annoyance, anger, resentment, tension, helplessness, sorrow, guilt, embarrassment, discouragement, or fear.

These feelings, largely unwelcome, can be called emotional distress. Emotional distress that occurs over and over again may suggest unresolved past or current problems. Some of these feelings will often go away on their own, others need to be managed using one strategy or another.

To know more about managing your body image and incontinence, ask yourself these questions:

1. What problems and challenges do you see your body image and incontinence creating in your life?
2. When faced with a problem you must do something about, what happens? What do you do? How do you feel? How often does the problem occur? How does it usually work out?
3. To whom do you turn if you need help?
4. What kinds of situations usually cause you emotional distress?
5. How has your body image and incontinence affected the people closest to you?

Effective Strategies

The goals of any coping strategy include preserving your emotional balance by managing the emotional distress caused by incontinence, preserving a satisfactory self-image despite incontinence, maintaining a sense of competence and mastery, preserving your relationships with family and friends, and dealing with any related medical treatment procedures.

What are the strategies or things people do to manage problems? Often people use more than one strategy, and each strategy is not necessarily good or bad. Coping can be seen as good when the approach you use is socially sanctioned or not reckless or harmful to yourself or others. It is important to understand exactly what your problem is if you hope to deal with it effectively. Some possible strategies may include:

- seeking more information,
- talking with others who have a similar problem,
- doing other things for distraction,
- using humor in describing the problem,
- accepting or finding something favorable about a problem situation,
- taking firm action based upon what you know about the problem, and
- considering feasible alternatives in future problem situations.

There is no secret formula for good coping that fits everyone. Coping is a skill that needs to be suited to the occasion. If one response or action better prepares a person for the next problem, then whatever works best is best for that individual. The important issues in any coping situation are: What are the results? Has emotional distress been reduced?

If coping is a skill, then it can be learned using some of the characteristics of individuals who are successful in coping with adversity. Research has found that individuals who cope well with other serious chronic illnesses such as diabetes and cancer seem to follow the guidelines in Box 1.

Individuals who manage well know the difference between being hopeless and powerless on one hand, and active and assertive on the other. Individuals who cope poorly tend to be rigid, overly compliant, and lack self-assertion. In fact, the difference between someone who copes well and someone who does not is the difference between resourcefulness and rigidity; between constructive optimism and pessimism where one expects a repeat of earlier frustrations. Those who self-manage or cope well confront problems, do what they can to solve them and reduce distress, and call upon available supports, including their own inner resources. They demand and yield selectively, anticipating realities, and knowing that not every problem can be solved every time. Nevertheless, problems can be solved more often through awareness and acceptance than through disavowal, avoidance, and denial. Individuals who cope poorly also mistake bravado or a habit of saying, "I can do it myself," for true independence. It often takes more courage to recognize a problem and accept help than to deny assistance and strive for unrealistic expectations. Indeed, those who cope poorly usually deny a great deal despite the existence of real problems, call upon wishful thinking, project blame onto others or onto themselves, or use overly passive approaches, waiting for something to be done for them by others.

Box 1. Coping Guidelines

1. Do not deny problems too often, too long.
2. Confront reality and take appropriate actions.
3. Focus on solutions to problems.
4. Be flexible and consider alternatives to problems.
5. Maintain open, honest, mutual communication with others who are important to you.
6. Seek and use constructive outside help.
7. Accept support when offered and needed, but seek independence whenever possible.
8. Keep up morale through self-reliance.
9. Develop a good self-concept, which is an important solution to any problem.

Managing Your Body Image and Reaction to Your Incontinence

Many people with incontinence view themselves as powerless and their bodies as "in control" of any given situation. When you feel powerless to control aversive events, you are more likely to experience anxiety, depression, and self-doubts. There are several strategies that you can use to regain control and to help strengthen a more positive body image. These strategies include constructive self-talk, avoiding negative thinking, assertiveness training, and progressive muscle relaxation. The more positive an image you have of your body, the more you will be able to manage your incontinence and enhance the quality of your life.

Self-Talk and Refuting Irrational Ideas

We all talk to ourselves. You might ask yourself what you want to eat for breakfast or what outfit you want to wear today. You also might tell yourself that you need to start a project today so you can meet next week's work deadline or prepare for a visit from family members. You might say to yourself that you look nice in an article of clothing. When your self-talk is realistic and supportive, you feel good about yourself and your self-image. When you talk critically to yourself (e.g., "my boss is not going to like the ideas I am going to present at the meeting" or "I think everyone knows that I leak"), you may experience self-doubt, sadness, and anxiety. Everyone has irrational thoughts at times; what is important is how we handle these thoughts.

Sometimes when you are feeling depressed or anxious, you might have racing thoughts such as "I am not attractive because I am incontinent" or "I am not going to get the promotion at work because my boss thinks that I smell." These racing thoughts are not only unproductive, but also result in extreme self-doubt.

There are two techniques that can be helpful for lowering your anxiety when you are having these types of racing thoughts. The first one is called *Thought Stopping*. With this technique, you are literally telling yourself to stop having these thoughts. Some people like to say the word "STOP!" in the middle of these racing thoughts, while others like to imagine large stop signs preventing the thoughts from continuing to race. An example of *Thought Stopping* is, "I am not going to get the promotion at work, because… STOP!" Stating the actual word "stop" or imaging that stop sign provides a distraction and a chance to regain control of your thoughts by finding an alternative way to talk to yourself at that moment – "Hey, don't be so hard on yourself!"

After you stop the thought and recognize that the thought is distressing and irrational, your next step is to modify the negative self-talk to a more neutral or positive tone. Once you have successfully stopped the thought, ask yourself how you would manage the situation if your thought came true. For example, what if you leaked while spending time with your friends? You might tell yourself that you always have some spare clothing with you and some items to help minimize any odor. After you have decided how you would manage the situation, you should examine the thought. For example, what evidence do you have that you are not attractive? A counterargument to the original thought can be, "I have been in several relationships, and my significant others have told me that I am attractive." Would your friends *really* stop spending time with you if you had an accident? What is the likelihood that this will happen? A counterargument to the original thought

Box 2. Thought Record Components

- First, write down the situation in which the thought occurred. Be as specific as possible. Include details such as location, who was with you, and the time of day.
- Second, write down what you felt (e.g., anger, sadness, guilt).
- Third, write down the self-talk that you experienced. Although writing down these thoughts can be hard, try to be as specific as you can. By being specific, you can go back to your Thought Record after the situation is over and understand what you were thinking.
- Fourth, change your irrational thought. Just like a detective interviewing a suspect, you need to ask yourself questions about your thoughts.

  1. **What evidence do I have that this is true?** Using the example from above – "What evidence do I have that I am not attractive?" – you might tell yourself that "friends often compliment me on my appearance, and I date regularly."

  2. **What is the likelihood that this will happen?** "What is the likelihood that I am unattractive? The likelihood is pretty low, because people can enjoy being in my presence, and they do not run away from me screaming. This was true before I developed incontinence and after!"

  3. **Am I over generalizing?** "Just because the new guy I just met did not want to go on a date with me does not mean that no one finds me attractive." "I have many friends who invite me to play cards with them, I over generalize when I think no one wants to spend time with me." "Just because I am uncomfortable being incontinent does not mean the whole world feels the same way." "Others have asked me out, I enjoy socializing, and others seem to enjoy being with me."

  4. **Am I thinking in extremes (black and white thinking)?** "Just because people are not telling me that I am extremely attractive every day, this does not mean that I am not attractive." "Because I had one accident at church does not mean I will always have trouble there."

  5. **Am I setting overly high standards for myself?** "While I wish I had not developed incontinence, it is not a sign of being imperfect, it is just a medical condition. I am vigilant about recognizing when I am incontinent, but sometimes I do not notice. I am going to be okay. This is a part of me, and my friends need to accept me for who I am. Being incontinent does not mean I am not attractive." How has your image changed since you became incontinent? Remember, it is *your interpretation of you* that has changed, and that can be challenged!

- Finally, use your newly created alternative self-talk statements. These alternative statements will not only be useful for you in the present but also for potential negative self-talk in the future.

can be "I have been incontinent when spending time with my friends, and they have been supportive of me," or "My friends understand that I am incontinent; if they do not want to spend time with me because of it, then maybe I need to increase my social circle to include people who are more understanding."

Developing a "Thought Record" can be helpful in not only recognizing negative thoughts and modifying them but also recognizing themes to these thoughts. (Thought Records generally have five components, which are exlained in detail in Box 2 on the previous page.)

The more you use Thought Records, the more you may notice that your <u>negative self-talk</u> shares a particular theme. By writing down and remembering your alternative self-talk statements, you will be able to counteract your negative self-talk statements more quickly.

Assertiveness Training

When you feel overwhelmed or unable to control your own body because of your medical condition, you may allow yourself to be bullied by others (e.g., sit quietly when someone mentions your frequent trips to the bathroom), or just be "cranky" all the time, unaware that you are angry about your incontinence and taking it out on others. When you are assertive, however, you are expressing your needs and feelings in a respectful manner. In today's society, assertiveness has become a negative word, and some people feel that assertiveness suggests acting pushy and putting your needs ahead of everyone else's. This is not so. When you are being assertive, you are expressing your needs without placing blame.

One way of being assertive is to use "I statements" in lieu of "You statements." For example, when you have arguments with loved ones, you might make a nonassertive, accusatory statement like, "You are inconsiderate because you never listen to me." A better way of making this statement would be, "I feel ignored when you play solitaire when I am talking with you." "I statements" are helpful because they allow you to express what you are feeling and they allow the other person to understand what behavior he or she is doing that is hurtful to you. When making "I statements," it is very important to be brief, maintain eye-contact, speak clearly and firmly (i.e., do not yell or whine), and set up a time to have the discussion that will be a convenient time for all of the involved parties. This allows the other person to see that you are being serious and that you want to improve the current situation.

Another important component to assertiveness training is telling the other person the benefits to changing the current situation. For example, you might tell your loved one that if he or she spends some time listening to you, you will be more likely to listen to his or her stories as well. Reminding your friend or family, "I greatly appreciate your understanding concerning my need to go to the restroom often; I don't like my incontinence any more than you, so please refrain from referring to it so often," is much more constructive than saying "Leave me alone," "You just don't understand," or "What's it to you." You will find that by taking an assertive stance you will feel better about how you interact with others and you will be rewarded with more positive responses. This then contributes to enhancing your self-image.

Anxiety Reduction and Progressive Muscle Relaxation

Progressive muscle relaxation is a useful technique for individuals experiencing depression, anxiety, chronic tension and pain, insomnia, and many other conditions. During relaxation you have a positive experience and receive feedback that you and your body are "one" and that even though you have an incontinence problem, you can work cooperatively with your own body to feel comfortable. This will help enhance your body image and see <u>your body as a friend ra</u>ther than part of you that you struggle with.

The concept behind progressive muscle relaxation is that experiencing a relaxed body while simultaneously feeling distressed is nearly impossible. Progressive muscle relaxation teaches an individual to learn to recognize bodily tension and how to relieve it.

During progressive muscle relaxation and most other relaxation exercises, an individual is typically lying down or sitting comfortably in a quiet room with his or her eyes closed. You might want to start the progressive muscle relaxation with some deep breathing. Deep breathing involves inhaling totally, holding this breath for a moment, and then exhaling slowly. You might also find that saying or thinking a "mantra," a relaxing thought or image, will help you become more relaxed. Some examples include: "Om," "relax," "my body is feeling heavy and warm," "I feel calm and relaxed," or "calm." You might want to create a comfortable image, a place where you feel safe, calm, and relaxed such as your favorite meadow, beach, or comfortable chair in the garden.

Once you are in a comfortable state, begin the progressive muscle relaxation exercise. During this exercise, you will tense individual muscle groups for five seconds and then relax the group for approximately thirty seconds. Some people find starting at one part of the body (e.g., the feet and legs) and working across the body (e.g., stomach, shoulder, arms, head, forehead, and jaw) an easy way to ensure working all of the muscle groups. This exercise takes approximately fifteen to twenty minutes to complete and should be performed one to two times every day in order to both master the technique and to receive the maximum benefit. Working to manage your tension is working cooperatively with your body and can enhance the image of your body as a comfortable part of your self, rather than as a part of you that causes distress.

Summary

Incontinence can play a major role in how you see yourself and how you experience your body image. The media constantly bombard us with images of "perfect people" who do not appear to have incontinence concerns. We are taught from a young age that we are supposed to be in control of our bladder and bowel, and if we cannot, then we have somehow failed. We have inaccurately learned that a positive body image does not involve moments of incontinence.

By accepting how your body functions you can work to regain a sense of mastery rather than an ongoing conflict with the image you have of your body. Using the techniques discussed in this chapter, such as constructive self-talk, avoiding negative thinking, assertiveness training, and progressive muscle relaxation, you can reshape your body image, learn to feel better about your body and yourself, and enhance management of your incontinence, thereby building on your own positive quality of life. You may have difficulty in exchanging old habits for new, more rewarding ones. Change might not always come easy, but it is important to continue to try to change your old habits into new ones. Patience, persistence, and time are important and needed ingredients. Don't give up. Your ability to increase control and make positive changes in coping with incontinence and body image is a tremendous power. Persistence and determination are important in developing this power.

Using the approaches in this chapter can assist you in changing your behavioral, emotional, and attitudinal reactions to body image concerns and incontinence.

Consider the following in implementing an approach to change:

1. Set specific goals for change regarding your body image and incontinence.
2. Understand how developmental and historical events (including familial, cultural, and social experiences) shape your attitudes about body image.
3. Use body and mind relaxation techniques to reduce anxiety and the physical results of stress by incorporating muscle relaxation, deep breathing, and positive self-talk to promote those skills that reinforce positive body image development.
4. Identify dysfunctional appearance assumptions or beliefs that influence body image and incontinence experiences. Examples include:
   - "If I could look just as I wish, my life would be much happier."
   - "Physically attractive continent people have it all!"
   - "The only way I could ever like my looks would be to change them."
5. Confront and modify thinking distortions in your incontinence-related thought processes and offer coping strategies for modifying them. Such distortions include comparing your appearance to others, perceiving attractiveness as an "all or nothing" comparison, or blaming any perceived physical unattractiveness on your urinary or fecal incontinence.

6. Develop coping strategies to alter avoidant behaviors related to body image and incontinence concerns. These may include avoiding sexual relations, exercising, or those *situations* (i.e., going to the beach or the gym) or *people* (i.e., physically attractive individuals) that tend to reinforce self-consciousness and body image distress.

7. Create increased experiences of mastery and pleasure by engaging in body-related activities with positive reinforcement, learning both coping skills and a problem-solving approach.

When Things Don't Come Easy

If you continue to have difficulty developing new, more rewarding ways of coping, consider consulting a professional. Professional help can introduce new situations that encourage the development of new behaviors, emotions, and attitudes that can improve the quality of your life.

Choosing a professional helper can seem like a difficult task. We recommend a licensed and board certified clinical health psychologist, psychiatrist, or social worker knowledgeable and experienced in medical psychology and, if possible, incontinence. Make inquiries about such professionals among fellow patients. Consult your medical doctors, university hospitals, or medical centers for recommendations of various professionals or groups dealing with incontinence or emotional reactions to medical problems.

Recommended Readings

If you are interested in reading further on the specific strategies for change discussed in this chapter, we recommend:

Alberti, Robert, and Michael Emmons. *Your Perfect Right: Assertiveness and Equality in Your Life and Relationships.* 8th ed. San Luis Obispo, CA: Impact Press, 2001.

Cash, Thomas F. *The Body Image Workbook: An Eight-Step Program for Learning to Like Your Looks.* 2d ed. Oakland, CA: New Harbinger Press, 2008.

My Best Kept Secret

TARA WILLSON, UK

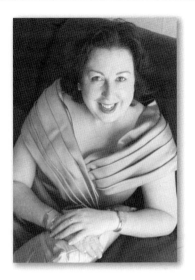

I'm going to tell you about the good, the bad, and the ugly. Why have I chosen this title? My disability is hidden, and for all my life I've struggled to keep my disability a secret. Many people in my life have no idea that I have a disability; but for me, it is a daily personal challenge. I come from an exceptional family of fighters and survivors in managing what we've got. No one will take the problem away, so we have to manage. My parents have had a lifetime of difficulty, not only with me, but also with my sister who was born with tuberous sclerosis and a severe learning disability. Even at age four, I knew I was in for a bumpy ride. My family has managed it – because we challenge things with a sense of humour and we all pull together.

I was born in 1966 with spina bifida. My spinal cord was fused to the spinal bones. Surgery was performed when I was 18 months old, releasing the spinal cord, but in the process damaging the nerves to the bladder and bowel – leaving me with double incontinence. However, even though I was under the care of one of the best children's hospitals in the world (Great Ormond Street Hospital, London) this information regarding my bowel and bladder was not given to my parents until I was five years old.

After I had lots of urinary infections the doctors at Great Ormond Street recommended that I have a urinary stoma operation. This procedure was irreversible at that time; my parents refused and demanded a second opinion in another hospital. Having heard and seen the positives of intermittent catheterisation, my mother persuaded the hospital to teach her.

I remember the first time that my mother was taught to catheterise me. The catheter was solid metal about eight inches long. I took one look at this strange metal object coming towards me and started crying. No one really sat me down and told me what the catheter was meant to do and why. No wonder I was physically sick. It was extremely traumatic. So mum came into my primary school at least once a day for about two years, and was catheterising me at least four times per day in total. It was all very noticeable: "Why does Tara's mum come into school every day?" I hated the taunting and the questions, not only by the other pupils, but also by the teachers.

Secondary school was looming and I didn't want my mum attending every day. So I taught myself to do intermittent self-catheterisation (ISC). There were some major disapproving comments by the medical profession, such as "How could a ten-year-old manage to do ISC?" But I did, and I flourished. Personally, I feel the earlier you can teach someone to catheterise, the better. It gives me such independence. It boosts my self-esteem, because I know that I may not leak as much urine, so this cuts out the panic regarding "Am I wet?" or "Do I smell?"

As for the other B (the bowel), I have always had constipation and little control, and I have to use laxatives. I was uncomfortable with laxative use because I had no control and would often have bowel accidents. So I have a neurogenic bladder and a bowel that is very unpredictable – two for the price of one.

School was emotionally difficult because no one was aware of the problem and it was a hard job constantly trying to hide it. I just wanted to be like everyone else. When I left school I was determined to get a job, and I did. I have always been employed.

So what does it mean, physically, emotionally, and financially, to have a hidden disability? I have always been aware of how different I am. Let's start with the equipment. I am the only person I know who goes on holiday with their luggage weighing less when they return than when they set off. Getting the right pads and having them delivered is a story in itself. My definition of happiness is the delivery of continence pads. Travelling around with a nine-inch catheter in its own make-up bag, spare pads, and spare clothes all means careful planning and thinking about the type of handbag I may need, while trying not to look conspicuous. Equipping myself now is not difficult; however, finding somewhere suitable to use the catheter and possibly change clothes can be hugely problematic. Imagine yourself trying to catheterise on a fast moving train or in a small toilet on a plane. Trying to sit/squat when in motion or attempting to change your clothes in a confined space needs skilled juggling! When in Egypt I learned in a matter of minutes how to catheterise standing up due to the less hygienic toilets I encountered.

I always like to know where toilets are, and plan any outing with military precision, including all social events. I would rarely consider walking in the countryside or attending an open-air music festival, because the toilets may have long queues and the hygiene levels are just not acceptable. All the thinking about and all the preparation for my incontinence often means not being able to act spontaneously, and can also be a barrier to living independently; but I won't give in.

On a day-to-day basis, I struggle emotionally to manage the unpredictability of being doubly incontinent. I work hard to appear a highly professional woman who doesn't smell, doesn't rustle like a Christmas present with the noise from the pads, and doesn't leave a trail of wet seats or have stained clothes. This struggle is day-in and day-out, but worse than that is the fear that an accident may occur.

The emotional costs, over the years, are very high and I've had to work very hard at building up my self-esteem. I do have my down days, as I'm sure everyone has. It's an ongoing battle that I know I have to face. When I look in a mirror I don't always see the same reflection back. I may not physically look different on the outside, but I know the inside is different. I don't have a label around my neck or a flashing light bulb above my head indicating that I'm different, but I certainly feel it. Personally, I feel that having a hidden disability is worse than having a visible one. If I was sitting in a wheelchair or using crutches people would obviously see there is a problem. With continence issues, by the time they see the signs (i.e., the wet clothes), it's too late.

So daily life revolves around knowing where the nearest toilet is. This means working at it every day to maintain dignity and respect for myself as a woman. As I've gotten older the second B (bowel) is now causing me more problems. I was referred to St. Mark's Hospital to see a gastroenterologist. I remember begging the consultant to remove my colon. Of course he said no. But he did offer me this amazing product, a new irrigation system that had come onto the market. It took me about nine months to get to grips with it, but perseverance pays off. It has changed my life. Just as my bowel problems were getting worse I started a new job that requires me to partially work outside. The nearest toilet is a twenty-minute walk away. How on earth was I going to hold down this job? The bowel irrigation system gives me security and assistance in clearing my bowel on a daily basis. I'm still learning what is "normal" for me, like no more onions, kiwi fruit, or processed bread. It's taken me several years of trial and effort, but I seem to be holding things together and carrying on.

Keeping my secret is difficult, as I don't want to broadcast my problems to a new friend or perhaps to a new employer. Getting and keeping a job, in my experience, can be difficult, but not impossible. However, I've learnt over time that it's best to inform your employer as you stand more of a chance of keeping your job.

It's all about trusting people with my secret. There are only a handful of close friends and family that I can trust. When it comes to meeting new people, especially men, I immediately panic. Relationships, especially intimacy, are an extremely difficult area for me. Some people I can't trust and some people just can't manage my disability.

As I've gotten older I've become more adept at keeping my best kept secret just that – secret! I look after my health better now and try to eat well, drink plenty, and respond extremely quickly to the first signs of a UTI (urinary tract infection). I'm in the process of reviewing my B&B situation with my consultants for any new inventions/processes. I am learning to manage/tolerate my hidden disability and for the first time in my life I am openly speaking about it.

You may associate "pee" with the bladder. The three Ps in my life are: I don't want peoples' pity, I want parity, and if parity is not forthcoming, I feel provocation.

Apart from my family and perhaps four close friends, I've had limited support from the medical profession or the specialist charities. In all aspects of my disability it is always me pushing for new information and knowledge. This is such a taboo subject that even family doctors struggle to talk about incontinence and can't refer me, because they don't seem to have much information. I have felt a burden, a failure, been humiliated, and am extremely frightened for my future. But nurses are the key to it all. Sensitivity and attitude are a necessity. I'm a really assertive woman, but I can crumble when I'm at the receiving end of patronizing and intimidating behaviours, particularly from hands-on staff. I do challenge such behaviour when I have the courage.

I have become involved in training health professionals about continence. When I do my presentations I ask delegates to think about how some behaviour and comments can make people with continence problems feel. One nurse said to me, "Oh I know exactly how you feel" – no, she doesn't; she has no idea! I want sensitively trained people.

I encourage nurses to try to speak openly about continence problems to their family and friends, and then when they reach the patient their fears and embarrassment will hopefully be diminished. They will then provide the patient with dignity, respect, and motivation, and support them not only physically, with catheters and pads, etc., but mentally. It strengthens us to know there is someone who will listen. If you really listened to us, we could manage so much better.

As to the future… I will continue to work hard and challenge my disability, continue to work full-time, and approach life with humour. I want to raise more awareness for the next generation coming along. I want to make it easier for people like myself, and press for more support. And finally, I want to release my Best Kept Secret!

I want to enlighten the world as to what it takes to live and deal with continence issues on a daily basis. Because we don't have a choice, we deserve the very best continence service our health service can provide.

There are three things I want you to take away from my words:

1. I want you to remember each person's continence difficulty is unique to that person. "One catheter doesn't fit all folks."

2. Clear, accurate information about all conditions and where to get help is vital.

3. In my experience as someone with long-term continence difficulties, I know that emotional support is absolutely essential.

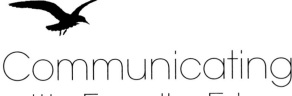

CHAPTER 6

Communicating with Family, Friends, and Colleagues

MARY RADTKE KLEIN, ANITA SALTMARCHE, RN, BScN, MHSc

EDITOR'S NOTE: We talk more easily these days about cancer, Alzheimer's disease, and erectile dysfunction. It still seems difficult, however, for many people to open a conversation about incontinence. Nonetheless, it's important. For some people incontinence can impact work life, social situations, and intimate relations. And then there are the accidents. This chapter proposes a strategy for separating fear and anticipated outcomes from your goals and desired outcomes. It proposes insights that help focus on and deal with facts in a conversation. It also offers ideas about finding the right words and trying out new approaches to conversations we too often find embarrassing.

Talking about personal health issues can range from being extremely easy to unbearably difficult. Recounting your recent golf game or work assignment may be effortless, but speaking about your incontinence or asking for emotional support in the face of an illness can provoke a lot of anxiety. If you feel uncomfortable about these conversations, we suggest that you set your emotions aside and remember that effective communication about important issues involving continence, is a process that generally takes a bit of time to learn and practice to improve, so be patient. A number of factors, such as the topic, our own self-talk, who you are speaking to, and previous experience, can all determine the difficulty of the conversation. With some forethought, these conversations may become easier than you think.

Some people who deal with incontinence choose to "pass" or "fly below the radar" using a mix of good planning, cautious strategies, and quick cover-ups. Although this can work, there is an emotional toll to maintaining a veil of silence. Talking about incontinence rarely means a tell-all disclosure. It's more likely that you will face a series of incremental decisions. Who do I need to tell? How much do I need to tell? What words do I use? What do I say to the people who look surprised when I jump up from the restaurant dinner table? How do I tell a romantic partner? What about the person whose house I'm staying at for the weekend? These decisions can be fraught with fear, often generated by the anticipatory stories we tell ourselves about how others will react. With thoughtful action, it's possible to move beyond this impasse of fear to more satisfying personal interactions and positive outcomes.

It is one thing to be able to manage the physical aspects of a misbehaving bowel or bladder; it's another matter to be able to talk about it. Some conversations are planned, some you might need to or want to initiate, and others are thrust upon you by a situation. In each case, there are some general principles presented in the chapter that should make these interactions easier and more effective.

Making the Conversation Easier

We all come with unique backgrounds. We have different experiences, beliefs, assumptions, values, and personalities. All of these shape you and may impact how and when you wish to communicate with others about your experience with incontinence. Perhaps you come from a family that is very open about personal issues. Maybe you have a few significant friends, but despite your closeness, you aren't in the habit of sharing personal or health information. Regardless of the kinds of relationships you have, the following principles should help you prepare for challenging conversations about incontinence… or any other sensitive issue for that matter.

Sorting Fear From Fact

All too often, we allow our assumptions and fears to influence what we say and how we say it. We focus on how we think someone will respond rather than on what it is we really want to say or request. For instance, if you believe someone will respond negatively, you may stall and then not bring up the matter at all. Or, you may use language that minimizes the importance of what you are saying or asking so your real request is not understood. When you formulate your words based on fear or anticipation of another's response, you often create a negative, self-fulfilling prophecy. Anticipating others' responses, or telling yourself how things will unfold before they actually occur, creates a fiction. Try thinking ahead about what is important to you, not what you anticipate the result will be. Try to be open to how a frank conversation will unfold.

Remind yourself that you cannot see the future, that you should not judge others through the lens of your worst fears. If you fail to do this, you limit the possibility of open communication because you have already decided how things are going to turn out. You also become less open to listening and hearing the other person's sincere response.

If your communication is based on your own well-thought-out goals and the outcomes you desire, you give the conversation a chance to unfold. You have said what was important to you. You need only to deal with the reality of the communication, not with what you imagined might happen, but what actually happened.

The Goal of the Conversation

As you are thinking about how to talk to someone about your problem with bladder or bowel control, ask yourself, "What is my goal or purpose in having this conversation? What do I want? What do I hope to accomplish by the end of this?" If you are not sure, then you might want to share your uncertainty:

"I want to tell you something about my circumstance, but I'm not sure if I just want you to know or if I want your help in some way. Maybe it will become clear as we talk."

Perhaps you want to just share some basic information, but you are not ready for a lengthy conversation:

"This is a bit difficult for me to talk about and I don't want to get into too many details, but I wanted you to know about something that I'm dealing with. It might explain a few things."

If you want the conversation to continue, you might say:

"…and I'd like your feedback… your opinion… your ideas about how I should handle this particular situation."

There is a big difference between simply asking someone to listen to you and asking for advice. By making the intention of your request clear, you avoid miscommunication and help to steer the conversation in the right direction.

"I need to get a few things off my chest about this condition. My talking about it, and just having you listen, would be a huge help."

"I'm having some issues getting into the washroom at home when I need to. I'd like us to sit down and decide together how we can manage to fix this."

Maybe you need some practical help to find products or services that will help you manage your symptoms, or you need to rearrange the bathroom schedule to make life a little easier. On the other hand, you may not want concrete help, but just a willing listener while you vent some frustrations. If you define your goals and make them clear in your conversation, you will begin to deal with the facts, rather than wander in the realm of fiction. Your conversations will become easier and more meaningful.

Choosing Your Words

It can be very difficult to find the right words to discuss your bladder or bowel. The topic does not tend to come up in most everyday conversations, so we have very little practice with it. The label "incontinence" itself can be difficult. It is a term that many are not even familiar with. Saying "I'm incontinent" also seems to imply a permanent, severe, or irreversible condition when in fact symptoms vary a lot. You may also be drawn into a long conversation trying to explain what "incontinence" means. It may be easier to talk about "leaking a little" or having an "uncooperative," "misbehaving," or "overactive" bladder or bowel. "An upset stomach" might work when a situation arises and you don't want to disclose the condition or provide any further explanation. A vague explanation may give you a quick, convenient cover.

Other words that come to mind sound like baby talk (pee, poo, poop) and still others are considered "dirty" or seen as swear words. Medical terms for bits of the body (urethra or rectum) are not common in everyday use and many people are unsure exactly what they refer to and so don't want to use them incorrectly or have to give a lecture to explain them. Bladder and bowel function are often the subject of teenage humor, and memories of this may also make adults reluctant to even consider talking about incontinence to anyone.

So, what words *should* you use? There is no simple answer. The point of talking about your incontinence is to communicate, in a way that you feel comfortable with and that others will understand. The main considerations are:

- Are the words you are using clearly understood by both yourself and the person you are talking to?
- Do both of you feel comfortable using these words?

The choice of words may depend partly on who you are talking to: friends, family, health care professionals, or colleagues. But also consider the individual. Certain family members may have clinical experience and health care providers will be quite OK with you not using anatomical terms. In fact, if you don't understand words they use, never feel reluctant about asking or checking that you have understood correctly. Clear communication is an important part of good health care.

If you feel like it is going to be difficult to talk about your bladder, bowel, or incontinence, plan what you will say in advance. Remember to ask yourself about your goal for the conversation. Then write the words down if that helps to think it through. Because we do not often talk about these things, it is naturally difficult to find the right words. Rehearsing can also help make you feel more comfortable and clear about what you want to communicate.

We live and connect by telling stories. If you have not told your story about incontinence to anyone before, it can be difficult the first time. Trying it first with a health care professional may be a good idea. If you are struggling to put it together verbally, try writing some key phrases out and handing them to the nurse or doctor when you are attempting to talk about your condition for the first time. It may make the process easier for both of you.

Introducing the Topic with Family, Friends, and Colleagues

Until recently, a colleague living with a congenital bowel malformation for more than forty years used the "secret agent" approach to "pass as normal." It required cautious strategies for blending in, quick cover-ups, and maintaining a code of silence. The result was a set of excellent how-to techniques (see Chapter 11, "Thriving Among the Thistles," for some specifics), well-crafted cover-up responses, a sharp mind for anticipation and problem solving and, all in all, a quite successful life. But, nonetheless, the emotional toll of carrying a secret was still considerable.

> " *When written in Chinese, the word crisis is composed of two characters. One represents danger and the other represents opportunity.* "
> —*John F. Kennedy*

You probably won't be confronted with an either/or decision to stay in the closet or totally come out. It's more likely that you'll face many small decisions about whether to talk about your incontinence or not. Do you want to introduce the topic, but don't know how to bring it up? Give some thought to your natural communication style and those to whom you're speaking. It may change how you wish to approach the topic. Directness and brevity might work:
"Did you know I have bladder incontinence?"

Maybe it would be better to preface the conversation with a few disclaimers:
"I know we aren't in the habit of talking about personal things, but I need to know that you don't mind discussing a personal health issue that's been on my mind."

The next time you are having a good laugh, an unexpected sneeze, or a hard cough, you might say:
"Oh gosh, I forgot to cross my legs. It's not an uncommon problem, but it sometimes catches me by surprise."

Is it your style to use humor, just to state the facts, or to tell stories when you communicate with others? Be honest with yourself and use whatever approach makes you feel most comfortable.

Help Them Help You

Frequently, the more information people have the better they are able to understand your situation and help you. This doesn't mean that you need to share every clinical detail and embarrassing experience. But it may be important to discuss how this condition came about and how it changed your life. Sharing some information puts curiosity to rest. It may explain why you can't lift up your grandchildren or go to a long church service or the theater. More importantly, people need to know what, if anything, you want from them and what they can do to help. It is a gift to be able to recognize what a friend needs and offer assistance without being asked, but very few of us can read minds – especially when someone may be trying to conceal a problem. Even the people who care most about you need to have information, permission, and some direction that lets them know how they can help and support you.

If you need emotional support, but you don't yet feel comfortable speaking to family and friends about these issues, there are other options. General and specific health-related support groups are available in health care settings and on the web. Within these supportive settings you will have the opportunity to share your experiences and feelings with others who are confronting the same symptoms and issues as you.

Work Colleagues

Sharing information about incontinence with your boss or work colleagues may be more difficult than sharing with family and friends. Your decision to disclose this information may be determined by whether or not you feel it is impacting your performance or ability to contribute at work. For instance, it may present a challenge if you need to travel for work. If your employer is trying to contain costs, he or she may not understand why you are unwilling to share accommodations with another colleague. If travelling to see clients is needed to build work relationships, you may seem uninterested if you always find reasons not to go. You may appear inflexible or not committed to the job. It may be that you need a colleague to cover your work when you need to make a sudden dash for the restroom. Others may need to understand why you make such frequent trips to the bathroom and that you are not shirking your job. It may be important to disclose the conditions you are dealing with and have work-related solutions to suggest:

"I think it is important for you to know something about me that relates to travelling for the company or being more actively involved with some work activities. I experience loss of bladder or bowel control. This has not affected my performance in other ways. But rather than travel frequently, I have scheduled/would like to schedule regular conference calls with my clients and am always available by phone when they need me. This would actually decrease company travel expenses. When I do attend conferences or meetings, however, I do need to book a single room."

Communicating in Those Embarrassing Situations

Personal conversations are one matter, but urgent incidents are another. They also call for planning, but less strategic thinking and more tactical response.

I have found that when one is embarrassed, usually the shortest way to get through it is to quit talking or thinking about it, and go do something else. —Abraham Lincoln

When It's Public

If you have paid attention to your body rhythms and stress level, your energy reserve, and your fluid intake and diet, you may find that you know when you might "get into trouble." Be aware and take extra precautions when you know you are vulnerable. When small incidents occur – and they will – there is no need to call attention to yourself or express regret. Excuse yourself and quietly attend to the matter. Others will take their cue from you. Those around you are usually far less observant of you and your condition than you might think and likely far more generous in their acceptance than you may give them credit for.

Have a set of tactical responses prepared, such as: "Excuse me, I'll be right back." "I have to take care of something; I'll be back in a couple of minutes." "Can you stop at the next place likely to have a restroom?" "I'll be back in a few minutes." Don't give yourself time to focus on your embarrassment or fear. Simply take charge and move through it. This is one of those rare times when it's better not to think too much. Do your thinking ahead of time.

Consider building a set of responses to questions you are afraid people will ask when you don't really want to open a conversation about the topic. You can choose to be the master of the non-answer or brush a question off with humor. Create and practice a few short, direct statements that provide information but don't invite follow-up questions: "Oh, I have a problem with my bladder. Did you say your brother Joe was coming into town next week? Didn't he just get back from China?"

If unexpected leakage requires an explanation or has involved someone else or their property directly, expect the best of them. Say what you need to directly and without making them embarrassed: "I need to stop at the next gas station." "Can we find a restroom right away?" "Oh, I'm sorry I've soiled your chair. If we can cover it for now, I will have it cleaned or repaired." "I have a problem with my bladder, will you excuse me." If you do excuse yourself and then return to an individual or group, try jumping back into the group's conversation or activity as if you haven't missed a beat. You save face and save everybody else from having to express their concern or exercise their curiosity. As quoted from Lincoln (above), "The shortest way to get through it is to quit talking or thinking about it ... do something ... ."

Finally, there you are at a party or after a movie and the bathrooms are occupied with a number of others waiting. How do you politely "jump the queue" or "cut in line"? Depending on your usual mode of communications, you may try:

"Sorry, but if I don't use the washroom next I will have an accident."

"Sorry, I have an overactive bladder, so I can't control it. Can I please go next?"
"I'm not feeling well and really need to use the washroom. Do you mind if I go next?"

When It's Very Personal

Who you confide in ought to be based on their need to know and your trust in their ability to accept and understand. If you are a houseguest or are sharing a hotel room, you may or may not feel it necessary to explain your need for periodic privacy, your longer bathroom stays, or the sealed bags in the garbage. Is your host or roommate accepting? Is she/he likely to be helpful, curious, or horrified? It makes a difference.

In a romantic relationship, it is probably unfair to confront a partner with big revelations at the very last moment. But when is the right moment? How much information is the right amount? There is little written to give us guidance, but here are a few thoughts.

As a relationship progresses, you are likely judging the character of your potential partner. You may want progress toward intimacy to be slow. If trust and affection builds, pick your time and place for "the talk." Project confidence. If you seem confident of yourself, you're partner is likely to feel confidence in the situation.

If intimacy is likely, your partner should not be surprised by an unannounced and unexpected sign of your condition: a brief, a collection bag, a physical difference. It's only fair to help your partner understand and anticipate the situation. Your communication might just mean disclosing a potential event – leakage or the need to follow a specific routine to assure good hygiene and comfort. You might begin by saying, "We are close enough that there's something you need to know. I have…" A medical diagnosis is often a good starting point; it keeps things a bit clinical, allows some discussion of the objective subject matter, and provides a way to ease into "so what does all that mean?" Let your partner know what to expect and that you know what you are doing. Then be gracious and provide this person you've come to care for with "an out" – a graceful way that allows them some time to think about this part of the relationship. It is likely your confidence will help the relationship move smoothly along.

In any of these communications you are likely to feel very vulnerable. Try to expect the best from others, but be gracious with those who don't have the capacity to be completely accepting.

In communication with others it's been suggested that you give some forethought to the conversations you might have, and then lead with confidence. Hopefully these examples and techniques will decrease your fear and negative anticipation of sharing your condition with others. Opening up the opportunity for this conversation with those who are close to you can be much more rewarding than you ever imagined.

38 Years of Incontinence

PAUL LAPORTE, CANADA

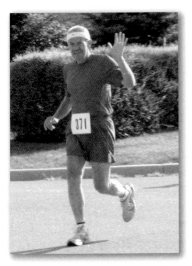

My name is Paul. I was born and raised in the 1950s in southern Ontario, Canada. My young life was uneventful and happy. There were certainly no continence issues in my early life. However, I had an asymptomatic tumour which was growing at the base of my spine and went undiscovered until age 22.

I remember one incident so well. I was at my grandfather's funeral and I had my first bladder control accident at the cemetery. That day was the beginning of my emotional fall caused by incontinence, in addition to my broken heart over losing my grandfather. Symptoms other than incontinence brought me to medical surveillance and surgery to remove the tumour.

While the surgery was successful in many respects, it left me with incontinence. The incontinence worsened quickly (within months), and by the time I was 25 incontinence was part of my life on a daily basis. At the time I was married to a wonderful woman. In many ways I attribute the break-up of my marriage to my withdrawal socially because of the incontinence.

My incontinence is restricted to urinary incontinence. In those early years I tried to cope by always checking out where the washrooms were. This was not a wise strategy, and my decision to become more of a recluse was taking hold. I always wore a diaper at night, for obvious reasons in light of sharing the bed with my mate. I was aware that diapers and plastic pants for adults were available, and I think mine were purchased through either the Eaton's or Sears' catalogue. My memory is vague; perhaps the diapers were custom made, either by my mate or one of her friends. What I definitely do remember is that there were no products in the 1970s comparable to what is marketed today.

Over time, I have become an expert on how my plumbing works. I don't leak urine constantly, although there are a few times when I do, which is most likely due to a urinary tract infection. For the most part my problems are associated with spasms and contractions, and when they happen the sphincter muscle is impaired enough that it cannot hold back the pressure, resulting in complete emptying of the bladder. This can be small quantities or larger quantities. If I am near or in a washroom there is a chance I can make it in time. I have found that, for me, activity plays a role in my coping ability, as does fitness and general health habits; but in those years these subjects were the furthest thing from my mind.

I have had my share of embarrassing "accidents," and while I can share those with just about anyone now, at the time they were devastating. I worked in an auto plant for four years and then I returned to college. During the very first month of school I had an accident in the cafeteria while having lunch, seated at a table with both male and female students. No one laughed that I could see, but inside I felt like just dying. There was no way I was going anywhere except home, and fortunately the friend who rode with me that morning tagged along – thankfully close behind me in order to minimize a gaping audience.

Right around this time my urologist introduced me to a McGuire Urinal. I remember the love/hate relationship I had with this product. It was difficult to put on, sometimes failed (if I had not applied it correctly), and was uncomfortable for prolonged wear. While I loved it during my school years, I also hated it because of how uncomfortable it was. It was made of a high-grade amber-colored rubber, and so were the straps that held the bag and top part in place. Daily, I had huge water blisters where the strapping dug in to my skin. Obviously, one could not wear shorts or participate in sporting activities, so I avoided those things. I continued to have accidents, but less frequently.

Prior to completing school, I was divorced. In retrospect, although devastated by the break-up, I can now appreciate that my incontinence and lack of coping abilities stood in the way of the outgoing lifestyle that we mutually enjoyed and that had bound us together. I had become reclusive, making every excuse imaginable to avoid the social limelight. This was my problem, not hers or even ours, and her perception of me not wanting to deal with it in a constructive way led to separation and ultimately divorce.

Now I was faced with new concerns. I did not want to resign myself to life as a hermit, and therefore the company of the opposite sex posed a whole new set of challenges regarding dealing with incontinence. I'm sure that many thought I was weird, or at least eccentric, because I was cautious about with whom, when, and where I would socialize (especially regarding the opposite sex). However, I soldiered on, hoping that my incontinence would not be discovered.

It was when I discovered advertisments for devices and products for incontinence that I realized there must be others like me. I wondered why I had not heard of this before, or met anyone like me. I frequented the University Medical Library, but there was little written regarding coping strategies or emotional assistance for dealing with the condition. I was living the lifestyle of a shut-in when I could, but I still had to go out and earn a living.

Then I met my current wife. Little did I know then that events would soon take a turn that would shape my life today. Initially, it was difficult because I did not know how I was going to break it to her without scaring her. The first planned weekend getaway was rapidly approaching. I wondered how I was going to deal with the wet bed, which was sure to happen. The first night away she woke up and caught me sitting in a chair and asked why I was not in bed. That night was the beginning for me of having someone listen to what I had been trying to get out of my mouth for so many years. It was also the beginning of a life-long up-hill struggle to recognize that incontinence can be merely an inconvenience, rather than complete devastation. I had longed for a family of my own, and now I had it, as she had two children. I credit my wife Jan for being there for me in the difficult situations that I would face.

Although in many respects I still felt rejections and failures, having a ready-made family made it time to become a provider. Because my primary method of coping with incontinence had been isolation, I still continued to fear and avoid the situations where my problem might be exposed. I gave up a promising career and promotion because I would have been required to travel. Fortunately, I was able to confide in my wife, and secure a less prestigious position with less remuneration. We both recognized that my talents were being wasted because of my inability to cope with incontinence.

During this time companies began marketing disposable absorbent products. I had, in addition to the McGuire Urinal, used diapers and plastic pants, and a waterproof pant with a snap-in liner. Carrying these products around posed its own issues; therefore it was a great boon to me to gain the option of disposable products. Equally impactful in my life was the discovery (through information tucked inside one of our product purchases) of the Simon Foundation in the USA. My wife encouraged me to make contact with them and to read their then-new (1985) book, *Managing Incontinence: A Guide to Living with Loss of Bladder Control.*

I learned so much from that book. I concluded that there was considerable work for me to do in regards to my own emotional status. I would have to force myself to socialize, or be encouraged by my wife to do so. I never had any social or emotional issues around her or around the children, who were eight and ten at that time. Indeed, my immediate family never raised any concerns at all regarding my altered lifestyle.

In November 1985, my wife and I made our first trip from Windsor, Canada to Chicago, Illinois so that I could attend the first self-help meeting ever held for those living with incontinence. I recall having a chilling fear, not knowing what to expect, or what would be expected of me. I left my wife at the hotel and made my way to the hospital classroom where we would meet. Although I was made to feel at ease, a comedy of errors was about to unfold which would make this first meeting truly memorable. There were several of us attending, all with various types of incontinence, all strangers to each other. Somehow we got locked into the meeting room when it was decided to close the door for privacy. The meeting was on a floor that the hospital closed up at the end of the business day, and although we had permission to use the venue, the hospital cleaning staff had not gotten the word; and so when the door was closed for our privacy, it locked – resulting in the most amazing "ice breaker" for an incontinence self-help group, especially since no one carried a cell phone back then and there was no phone in the room with which to call someone to let us out.

Aside from the trauma of being locked in and the relief of the rescue, my eyes were opened wide by what I saw and heard that evening. Here were people my age, and younger and older, both men and women, all learning how to cope. I left that meeting vowing to myself that I would work through my own insecurities. I remember that night lying awake in the hotel with my wife, who had this look of disbelief on her face. We had previously rarely talked about managing incontinence, and here we were talking about all the ways that I had to do things differently.

From that day on my connection with the Simon Foundation solidified, as did the connection with my inner self. The help I was getting in many ways created a re-birth of who I should have been had my earlier years not derailed my mindset into the depressed and helpless state that took so many years of my life. Finally I was able to begin living life in a more positive way, helped enormously by knowing that I was no longer alone.

Several conversations and many more trips to Chicago gave me the strength and confidence to manage my incontinence so that I could think of it as an inconvenience rather than a disability. I was asked if I would be willing to tell my story to the media. The Foundation was embarking upon a public relations campaign to get the message out that incontinence could be treated and managed. So I put forth a brave face and appeared in the media in Detroit, Philadelphia, and Pittsburgh. Even a bit of my story appeared in *Time* magazine. It did not stop there, either, as the Simon Foundation was expanding into Canada, and I was on the first Board of Directors of Simon Canada, now the Canadian Continence Foundation.

I credit my wife and the Simon Foundation directly for how I grew into a mature, confident, and educated man. Today I work for the Ontario Ministry of Labour and provide representation for injured and disabled workers in the Province of Ontario. I specialize in occupational disease claims, and yes I have represented workers with incontinence. I was even successful in representing a lady who damaged her pre-existing bladder condition by lifting things at work.

Today, I am more incontinent than ever, but it does not stop me from pursuing whatever I want from life. I would have never thought that I would be where I am today. When I turned fifty, I changed my life for the better. I shed about ninety pounds, quit a nasty smoking habit, and took up running. In fact, together with my daughter I have done a couple of marathons and several half-marathons and other races. I leak more than ever, but it does not prevent me from competing.

I would be remiss if I did not admit that I have been embarrassed in the near past, and expect that I will be again in the future. Yet nearly 38 years have slipped by, and I have never been subjected to one ill comment from anyone about my incontinence. I know now that no one needs to suffer alone with the condition. There is help for the asking.

CHAPTER 7

Communicating with Your Health Care Professional

ANITA SALTMARCHE, RN, BScN, MHSc

EDITOR'S NOTE: Incontinence is fundamentally a medical issue. Early assessment and realistic treatment options depend upon clear and effective communication. Between patient embarrassment and busy medical practices, however, it is easy for incontinence to get less attention than it deserves. The result can lead to increased loss of function and diminished quality of life.

This chapter encourages early and effective conversations with health care professionals. It explores ways to approach these conversations and to provide health professionals with necessary information. From being prepared for an appointment to being appropriately assertive about your needs, the suggestions help you avoid vague language in describing your symptoms. There are reminders to sort emotions from symptoms while remembering to be concrete about the impact incontinence has on your daily life. Recommendations are suggested for an effective patient-professional dialogue during a visit, clarifying what has been said, follow-up, and second opinions if the outcome of the visit seems unsatisfactory.

When something of a delicate nature needs to be shared in detail, especially when it relates to personal matters like your health, finding the right words, tone, and attitude to express it can be challenging, regardless of who you are speaking to. Loss of bladder or bowel control – incontinence – can affect your physical, psychological, and social well-being and given its complex impact, it can be very difficult to put together the right words to communicate your concerns to your doctor or maybe even to yourself. With some forethought, however, the conversation with your health professional may be easier than you think.

As a means of protecting ourselves, we frequently create barriers around incontinence, due to its private and often seemingly embarrassing nature. If you break through these barriers and decide to come out of the closet, you will become aware of a number of important realizations. You are not alone: millions of others experience incontinence. There are many resources available to assist you. Generally, people are very supportive and understanding when you share sensitive information.

When we speak about communicating we most often think about the dialogue between two individuals. But we also need to think about the dialogue that goes on in our own heads, referred to as "self-talk." We often are not aware of how limiting our own self-talk can be. This self-talk can be negative, neutral, or positive. Unfortunately, it is frequently negative, feeding our fears. This negative self-talk can significantly alter how we speak to others and may even color how we receive or hear what others are saying to us.

Speaking with family, friends, or colleagues can be quite different from talking with your health care professional. This chapter will provide you with useful tools to improve your communication about your bladder or bowel control concerns. Open, honest communication is the key to all strong relationships.

Advance preparation for a difficult conversation, especially for emotional topics, can alleviate much of the associated stress, as well as clarify your goal and anticipated outcomes. The preparation increases the likelihood of having a clear, concise, meaningful interaction in which you are understood and receive the desired results.

Note: It is important that you have or have had a thorough assessment and workup and that all potential treatment options are explored. Since this book is written for those who cannot at present have their incontinence cured, it is assumed that you have already discussed your experience with incontinence with your doctor. If you have discussed the issue with your doctor and nothing more can be done medically, it is still important to periodically acknowledge that the condition does negatively impact your life and ask whether there is anything new that may assist you. If you read this section and feel you may not have clearly communicated your condition or were not heard, then review the chapter and book an appointment.

"See your doctor sooner!"

During the best of times, a trip to the doctor's office usually doesn't fall under our list of favorite things to do. Certain fears may emerge when we think of going in for an appointment:

What if he thinks I'm exaggerating my symptoms?
She won't find this important.
As soon as I enter the examining room, my mind goes blank!

When it comes to talking about incontinence with your doctor, a host of other worries may join in with all of the regulars:

How can I talk about something so private and embarrassing?
What if I get emotional when I try to talk about my bladder problems?
What if he shrugs it off? What if it's just a normal part of aging?

These worries were voiced by women participating in a study on incontinence. Many of them admitted to putting off the doctor's visit for years, waiting until their incontinence became almost unmanageable. When asked if they had any advice to pass on to others dealing with the same problem, many emphatically said: "See your doctor sooner!"

"I didn't realize it was such a problem for them."

In the second half of this research, family doctors and specialists (urologists and gynecologists) were interviewed about their interactions with patients who experienced incontinence. The following doctor reactions may provide some insight into behaviors we may sometimes encounter when we speak to doctors or other health care providers:

Often they (my patients) mention the issue, but it is just as I am walking out the door, so it must not be very important.

Well, in the scheme of things, such as heart disease or high blood pressure, it isn't very serious.

Well it isn't cancer! When you deal with another patient a few minutes earlier and have to discuss their limited treatment options and their likelihood of survival, it is difficult to see incontinence as significant.

Incontinence isn't going to kill them.

There isn't time to deal with three or four symptoms or health conditions in one appointment. We are always behind schedule.

When doctors were faced with quotes demonstrating how anxious individuals were to discuss their incontinence with their health care providers, the vast majority of the doctors were quite surprised. Most admitted they did not routinely ask about incontinence, but most were more than willing to address it if it was brought up. None of the doctors said that they were uncomfortable dealing with the issue.

The doctors acknowledged that it was difficult to remain current with all of the medical developments, especially considering the number of conditions they encounter daily. Some did not feel adequately prepared to address incontinence, but were willing to refer to a specialist for further workup when required.

These results further support other research which indicates that clients and doctors view incontinence from different perspectives which may contribute to misunderstandings and miscommunications between the two groups. Understanding the different viewpoints can assist in clarifying communications.

Patient Responsibilities

If you have ever attempted to describe your incontinence symptoms to your health care provider, you may recognize one of these scenarios:

Doctor: *So is that everything?*

Patient: *Yes, yes. Well, to tell the truth, I have been having some problems making it to the washroom on time. Sometimes I really have to rush. But it's no big deal. We can talk about it some other time. Goodbye!*

Doctor: *What brings you here today?*

Patient: *Well, one thing is when my feet are cold I have to use the washroom… and I've stopped taking dance classes, and I don't go to church any more. And… I don't know… uhhh… never mind about that.*

Embarrassment or not wanting to feel like a "nuisance" may account for not communicating directly about your incontinence. But that kind of hesitant presentation will give the doctor the impression that the symptom is not important, and therefore does not need to be explored any further.

Many people take the spontaneous approach to conversing with their doctor or nurse. Whatever pops into their heads when they enter the examination room is what they say. One problem with taking this route is that you are certainly not in control of the outcome of the appointment.

The preceding examples may seem exaggerated, but it is often the case that patients who do not have a clear goal for the communication during an appointment make it almost impossible for the doctor to do his or her job well. Your responsibility as a patient is to help your doctor help you.

It is important that you not only describe the loss of bladder or bowel control symptoms, such as frequency, amount, or consistency of leakage, but also how it affects your day-to-day activities and quality of life. It is easier to understand how important a condition is when both the medical information and its impact are presented clearly. This will greatly increase the likelihood that you will receive the best possible health care.

A central shift is beginning to take place in health care fields. A new recognition of the importance of the patient as an active participant in his or her own health is taking hold of medical practice and health care in general. Research in this area has shown that patients who develop working relationships with their doctors and other health care professionals are not only happier with their care, but actually receive better care and better results.

As a patient, it is vital for you to recognize that the patient-doctor relationship is not entirely in the hands of the doctor. Studies have shown that despite their awareness that patients are hesitant to speak about incontinence, health care providers rarely prompt their patients into discussing these symptoms. If your doctor does not ask and you hesitate to disclose your symptoms, how are you going to access clinical assessment, treatment options, practical information, and the support you need? The rest of this chapter will focus on some practical solutions to make the most of each appointment you have with a health care professional and to avoid the wasting of an opportunity when you speak to your health care professional.

Before the Visit

Gathering Information

The more information health care providers have about your condition, the more seriously they will view the situation. That being said, good communication with your doctor begins with a plan. It is important to prepare by learning as much as you can about your bladder/bowel control problem. You can do this effectively by keeping a diary or log to collect and present relevant information. Then, explore ways of expressing this information to your doctor. If you are able to provide specific information and ask clear questions, you will make the most of the time you have with him or her. Together, the two of you can work toward finding a solution that works for you.

Bladder Chart

Date/time	What happened?	Amount of leakage	I made it to the toilet
Monday 3:30 PM	Carrying box to basement – little spurt of urine when I put box down	Small amount	No
Tuesday 1:00 PM	Strong urge while finishing lunch	Wet pants but didn't soak through to outer clothing	No
Wednesday			
Thursday			

Here is a list of information that your health care provider will need to know:

1. The frequency and intensity of warnings, urges, and/or accidents. Along with the record, write down any concerns that you would like to discuss. It might be a good idea to make a *bladder and/or bowel chart* to bring in with you when you see the doctor. This will provide needed information, as well as indicate that you expect your condition to be taken seriously. (Please see bladder chart on previous page.)

2. Make a list of the medications you are currently taking or have recently taken, including over-the-counter drugs (i.e. Tylenol, Advil) and herbal supplements. If this is not your regular doctor, it may be helpful to bring the medications in with you to the appointment.

3. Also, be prepared to answer some of the following questions:

   Have you had children? How long ago? What type of births did you have?
   Have you reached menopause? How long ago?
   Have you recently been injured?
   Have you had prostate surgery?
   Have you had any operations? What were they for?
   Do you have pain when you use the toilet?
   Do you have: cancer, arthritis, diabetes, depression, spinal cord injury, etc.?
   Do you have to get up at night to empty your bladder or bowels? If so, how frequently?
   Do you have hesitancy in starting your stream or decreased flow of your urine?
   What is your usual bowel function: loose, constipation, fluctuating between these?
   Amount of leakage with an accident?

Describing the Impact on Your Life

Before you can describe the impact of your symptoms to your health care provider, it is important to be aware of it yourself. Many individuals underestimate the impact that incontinence has on their lives. Spend some time thinking about the "used to's" in your day-to-day life. I used to... volunteer, go to the theater, go out with my friends...

Think about whether these statements, expressed by others who have bladder control problems, apply to your situation:

I often decide not to leave the house because of a potential accident.
I need to be prepared and carry an extra set of clothes at all times.
I can't laugh without leaking all over my pants or skirt.
Before I can confidently leave home, I need to map out exactly where the washrooms are.
I never wear anything other than dark clothes, just in case.
I used to love going on hikes with my family.
There is this constant fear of an unexpected accident.

One study found that over eighty percent of the individuals interviewed curtailed their social activities because of their bladder or bowel control problems. These activities ranged from participating in sports, to engaging in intercourse with their partners, to coughing or even laughing.

These are all examples of altered behavior and activities due to incontinence. Think about these and other ways that incontinence has affected your life. This is the first step to learning how to effectively communicate this problem with your doctor. Begin thinking about the things you used to do, coping strategies and adaptations you have made to live with the problem. It may be helpful to write down all of the ways incontinence has affected your life. Try to be as honest, as detailed, and as specific as possible.

Describing Your Symptoms Effectively

Responses to bladder or bowel control problems can range from complete acceptance to extreme distress. Just as every individual has his or her own communication style, we also respond to health problems in different ways. Some people cannot help but express their symptoms with strong emotion:

My life is over. I cannot believe this has happened to me. It affects my sleep, activities, emotions, everything.

Others tend to take the stoic approach, accept their loss of control, and move on without looking for possible solutions:

This is a normal condition that isn't too bad. There's no need to bother anyone else about this problem.

As different as these responses are, they make it equally difficult for a doctor to know exactly what a patient is looking for during a visit. The words you choose when you describe symptoms are very important, because they give clues to assist your doctor in determining the degree of impairment and making a correct diagnosis. This section will provide insight into how to communicate information in a way that will cause a doctor to address your condition in a serious manner, so that together you can move toward solutions that work for you.

Avoid Underestimating the Impact of Your Symptoms

I know this is just a normal part of being a woman, but…
I thought I'd mention it to you, but it's really nothing to worry about…
I have to stop at almost every hole on the golf course because of my urgency, but all the guys do, so I guess its not important.

If you followed the earlier advice and have written down the ways in which your bowel or bladder control problems have impacted your day-to-day life, look at these descriptions again and check for words or phrases that minimize the effect of your symptoms or state your concerns using apologetic words. Cross these words out. If you need to, re-write the list using clear and direct statements that honestly describe the changes that have occurred due to incontinence:

My constant urges to use the washroom make it very difficult for me to participate in my social activities. As a result, I feel cut off from the things that are important to me in my life, like my grandchildren, friends and family… and I would like to work toward a solution to this problem.

I find I can't sit through a movie, carry regular bags of groceries, or attend a long work meeting without excusing myself several times…

Avoid Vague Descriptions

Being vague in your descriptions of your symptoms does not help your doctor, nurse, or other health care provider gain a clear understanding of the issue and, in turn, will not help you access the information you need. Some examples of vague descriptions of symptoms include:

I have to go more often than I'd like.

I sometimes have a problem making it to the bathroom.

I don't have the same bladder control anymore.

This approach may prevent your doctor from doing his or her job properly. Your health care practitioner may not have time to ask you many follow-up questions to get the information they need.

It is important, when thinking over the list of questions your doctor may ask you, to be able to answer them as clearly and specifically as possible. Here are possible ways to reword the statements above:

Two years ago, I was going to the washroom 6-8 times a day. Now, I go at least 16 times a day and feel the urge to go even more than that.

Last week, there were four separate incidents where I had an accident before I made it to the washroom.

Separate Your Symptoms From Your Emotional Responses to Them

Distress or embarrassment may be a natural response to the stresses of living with incontinence, but they may also be a barrier to accessing the kinds of treatments that can help you.

It is only natural to take your health issues personally, for they affect your life in ways that only you are aware. Generally speaking, although you may feel your condition is private and personal, to the doctor it is a symptom that needs to be explored, a medical issue. Health professionals do not make personal judgments about incontinence or get embarrassed.

For the sake of effective communication, realize that your doctor or nurse understands your symptoms in an entirely different way than you do. Each issue is, for them, a challenge to be overcome or a puzzle to be solved. Health care providers often adopt a "find it and fix it" approach to health problems. Because of this, the language you choose to use will be interpreted by your health care team in a unique way. Take a look at the differences between the communication styles of these two patients: The distressed patient may feel the problem is so complex and overwhelming that he or she doesn't know where to begin. The effective patient is someone who understands that his or her health care team will listen to a direct explanation and help to find a solution. Adopting a more pragmatic approach to your symptoms may be a challenge at first, but it will most likely result in better care for you.

During the Visit

Ineffective Communication
The patient says:
I am so humiliated! I can't leave my house! I don't participate in anything any more.
The doctor hears:
Is she depressed, needing medication or counseling?

Effective Communication
The patient says:
My bladder control problems are significantly affecting the quality of my life. I'm interested in hearing about treatment options.
The doctor hears:
Incontinence needs to be investigated. Once we know the type of incontinence, options can be discussed.

It is not only patients who sometimes minimize symptoms or offer vague explanations. This section will provide you with potential responses to health care professionals when they are too vague or underestimate your concerns.

What to Do if Your Health Care Professional Underestimates Your Concern
How is a patient supposed to respond when they are faced with this reaction from their doctor?
Don't worry. It's nothing serious.
Just go more often.
It could be worse… it's not a recurrence of your prostate cancer.

Your health provider may be responding in this way for a number of reasons. Ask yourself if your doctor is responding to your own interpretation of your symptoms. If you believe this is the case, reiterate your concerns including your symptoms and their effect on your quality of life. See if it evokes a better response from your doctor. The clarity and directness with which you state and even restate your position indicates its relevance to you and the seriousness with which you want the doctor to respond to your issue.

Here is one way you could redirect your doctor back to the topic at hand:
You may have misunderstood me. I meant to say that I am experiencing frequent and intense urges to use the washroom, and it sometimes causes pain. I am interested in learning more about available treatment options.

A second reason your health care provider may underestimate your concerns is due to the time constraints of the appointment. If your doctor doesn't have the time to address your condition properly given the time scheduled for the appointment, do not hesitate to raise this issue. It is in your best interest to ask if you should schedule another appointment to talk about it:
You look very busy. Should I schedule another appointment so we can talk about this further? I'd rather schedule another appointment so we can really address this issue.

Finally, there is the possibility that your health care provider doesn't have the training or knowledge about incontinence to adequately help you. If you get this impression, it is worthwhile to ask if there is someone else he or she can refer you to:
Is there a medical expert that specializes in incontinence to whom I can be referred?

Most health care professionals would be pleased to direct you to someone who can help you sort out the treatment options that would work best for your condition. To reiterate, the goal of your health care team is to "find it and fix it," and if they lack the resources to do this themselves, they will probably know someone who can help. Keep in mind that you have as much responsibility as your health care provider to ensure that you get the care you desire and deserve. If your health care coverage requires a referral in order to consult a specialist (a urologist or urogynecologist), don't hesitate to be assertive about asking to see a specialist. The application of special expertise may be necessary to establish a definitive diagnosis and evaluate the latest medical interventions.

Asking and Answering Questions
If your doctor asks you further questions, it is because he or she needs more information to understand your condition and how to best help you. Try your best to answer your doctor's questions as honestly and as clearly as possible, even if you find them embarrassing:
Does the incontinence interfere with your sexual activity?

Sometimes doctors tend to fall into technical language that is hard for us to understand, or may rush through explanations that are important for you to understand. If you have any questions for your doctor, ask them. If you do not understand the answers you receive, do not hesitate to ask again. If the answer is still not clear, ask your health care provider to explain it to you in a different way:

I'm sorry, but I did not understand everything you just said. Would you mind explaining it again? Can you explain it more slowly?

Do you have any printed information about this?

Would you explain how this medication will help me? Can it cause side effects?

I don't really understand the treatment plan. Can we please discuss the plan and my options?

One very effective way of making sure you understand what your doctor has said is to say it back to him in your own words. *Do I have this right, you said...* This will not only show your doctor that you are listening and hearing what he has said, but it will also provide him the chance to clear up any misinterpretations. Other questions you should never hesitate to ask are:

Is there anything more that can be done to help me regain any of the activities I have had to give up because of the incontinence?

Is there any way for my family to help me?

Who can I talk to about my emotional or social concerns?

Above all, don't hesitate to voice your concerns about side effects of various treatments, or to ask if alternative treatment options are available. This is your time. Don't regret how you spent this time, wishing you had asked this question or that.

On Second Opinions

If you sense that your doctor may be under-informed about incontinence and your specific control issues, and doesn't have all of the answers to your questions, don't assume that your questions cannot be answered. Family practice doctors may not have received in-depth training in conditions that cause incontinence. There may be other members of your health care team who are able to help.

If you are referred to another doctor or specialist, it is important to realize that it is not because you doctor doesn't care about your needs: quite the opposite. He or she is working to find you the help you need and deserve. You might even consider getting a second opinion without prompting, in order to better understand all of your options. Each health care system is different. You may or may not need a referral from your family doctor to access a medical specialist. In some countries there are nurse continence advisors available and self referral may be an option.

If you have product questions, or have physical or emotional needs, remember, there are other health care professionals, such as nurses, social workers, and psychologists with unique and important skills. These individuals are qualified to help you cope with the various aspects of incontinence. Additionally, the Simon Foundation for Continence as well as other continence foundations worldwide have excellent websites and resources available to increase your knowledge about the condition, potential treatment options, and helpful product advice in order for you to live the fullest life possible in spite of your leakage problems.

After the Visit

If you feel as though the treatment options offered to you are not working, do not hesitate to schedule a follow-up visit to discuss what the next alternative may be.

In summary, if your goal is to achieve the best quality of life while living with incontinence, mastering the art of successful communication is an important first step. When approaching your family, friends, or health care providers, keep in mind that you have your own beliefs and assumptions about incontinence, and so do they. Have realistic expectations about what you hope to accomplish. But also realize that sharing this private part of your life with those who are closest to you will often strengthen your relationships. As well, and importantly, it may relieve the burden of secrecy. Thinking and fretting about sharing your experience with incontinence is often much worse than actually speaking about it. Most people are not only receptive and supportive to the disclosure of sensitive information; they can be of great assistance.

Your health care providers may be able to offer a wealth of information on treatment options and support groups available to you. They may also be able to rule out any underlying cause, or refer you to a specialist who can. When speaking to your health care providers, realize that your good health is a goal you both share. The benefits that will come when you decide to share your condition far outweigh the possible embarrassment it may initially cause. Effective communication often begins with a plan. If you know what you're looking for, you are much closer to achieving it. Take the step and experience the positive outcomes.

My Life Revolved
Around My Bladder

ELAINE, CANADA

The birth of my third child (let's call him Joey) in 1984, when I was 31, did not go smoothly. After twelve hours in the maternity ward, my doctor was startled to run into me. The seasoned maternity nurse had not notified him I was there, because she did not believe me when I said that my water had broken. By then an infection had settled in and both Joey and I were on intravenous antibiotics for several days. The nurse overseeing my labor insisted the doctors would eventually realize a Caesarian was necessary. As my labor progressed my doctor was joined by a team of obstetricians until one said he thought he could (and did) deliver Joey by forceps.

I was surprised by how thin and long Joey was compared to my previous chubby babies. But at 9lbs. 11oz., he was no lightweight. The doctor giggled as he extended the graph on which he was to record his length and the circumference of his head, both of which were greater than what was supposed to be the 100th percentile. Other parents did a double take as I walked past with the baby and my sister broke out laughing, saying name tags were hardly necessary, when she looked into the nursery and saw a group of cute newborns and one baby whose head was twice the size of the others. Everyone agreed that they had not seen a healthy newborn with such a large head.

As the epidural anesthetic wore off, urine started to run out of me uncontrollably. When we came home I found the maternity pads would not hold the urine, which just seemed to run steadily from my bladder. The baby was colicky and cried constantly, and I cried constantly because I could not stop the urine. My doctor examined me and then stated: "Well it is not the worst prolapse I have ever seen." When I asked what could be done he suggested that if I continued the Kegel exercises and lost the baby fat, it might help.

I got my weight down to 132 pounds, which was quite acceptable for my 5'5" frame. I resided in a jurisdiction where all the medical services were covered, and I enrolled in a paid service where a nurse attended weekly to oversee the Kegel exercises with a biofeedback machine. Eventually there were gaps in the day without urine leakage, but I could not ever go without pads. Standing, walking, sitting down, reaching – they all caused urine to run.

I didn't know how I could go out in public. When I went back to work (I was a partner in a large law firm) I had to wear more than one pad at a time and carry a big bag to change them frequently during the day (I was too embarrassed to buy incontinence pads). I carried an extra pair of underwear; I was terrified about smell. As a child I had gone to a school with a handicapped girl who smelled of urine and I feared that it was the same for me. As my tissues were bathed in urine at all times, I had chronic vaginal irritations and took to applying Vaseline. I watched constantly to determine where bathrooms were. When I arrived at someone's house I immediately went to the bathroom, and of course had to go before we left.

Disposing of the used pads was a problem. Not everyone has a garbage basket in their bathroom. I had to carry a bag in my purse to seal in the wet pads. I showered more than one time a day. I recall once when we were at a motel we just could not get enough towels because I showered so frequently.

My life revolved around my bladder. When my husband and I separated many years later he referred to the fact that he had had to deal with the incontinence. When he told me of his desire to separate he indicated that he wanted "to stay young" while I was "determined to get old." When asked for particulars one of the things he mentioned was my (by then cured) incontinence. He told a professional dealing with us that I had "urinary incontinence" as if that was all anyone needed to know to explain our impending divorce.

I did report the incontinence, in fact constantly, to my doctor who eventually referred me to a specialist – a urologist. The urologist carefully explained to me, as if I was cognitively impaired, that urologists were the male equivalent of gynecologists. When I reported this back to my primary doctor he sought out someone who had expressed an interest in treating women. This individual explained that mothers often developed incontinence because they went to the bathroom every time they got up with the baby. I called this the reverse toilet training theory. Hanging around with un-toilet-trained children caused mothers to regress.

A third doctor to whom I was referred talked about surgeries that could be done, but stated that they often failed and only worked temporarily. When I asked how long the surgery would work he said maybe two years.

I just didn't accept that this was all that could be done. So I changed my primary doctor in order to get into another referral group. By then I had gained weight and was about 150 pounds, and thus I was told that my weight was to blame. Pointing out that the problem was worse at 132 pounds was received with a blank face.

At one point I was even referred to a neurologist, who wrote back it wasn't a neurological problem. At another point I was referred to a hospital that treated spinal cord injuries. They tested me exhaustively and really couldn't see the problem; after all, they dealt with people who couldn't walk.

Through all this I developed depression and was on antidepressants, which allowed the next urologist to state that clearly I had more serious problems than incontinence. When I complained about how much incontinence bothered me, I clearly had emotional problems, but when I didn't mention it at all, then of course it must not be a serious issue for me.

When I was told that it was not life threatening, I pointed out that my acne wasn't either, but my dermatologist still was aggressively treating it. This doctor pointed out that acne was very different as it was visible.

I read a couple of books that were related to womens' health issues and tried to discuss what they had to say about incontinence. But clearly anyone who would buy a book written for a popular audience and then refer to it when consulting with a specialist, was of course a little nuts; or at least that was the message conveyed by their condescension.

I saw eleven specialists; those who thought that there might be a surgery available said that it was very rarely successful, and when it was, it "wore off" in a few years and would definitely not work for someone who was overweight.

I still cringe with embarrassment when I think about the day someone in my office noticed that my office seat was urine stained. I withdrew generally from social situations. I just went to work and came home and looked after the kids. Eventually I gave up my practice as a lawyer.

In time I also developed chronic cystitis – which I do not accept was completely unrelated – and in 1995 was referred to Dr. Sender Herschorn. By this time I think I weighed about 180 pounds – as did eleven-year-old Joey who was close to six feet, shaving, and playing rugby. Dr. Herschorn indicated that the chronic cystitis was an intractable problem but why, he wondered, had I never done anything about the incontinence? He said they could do a rather simple surgery that was quite successful in reversing stress incontinence. If someone had suggested this surgery ten years earlier I would have dropped everything to do it right then and there, but having been told so many times that surgery was rarely successful I could not get excited about it. However, I went ahead anyway.

I will never forget the day that I woke up from the surgery, and for the first time in eleven years and three months woke up with a dry pubic area. The leak was plugged. It felt like a miracle. I was bone dry. The surgery was 100% successful. When the doctor came around and asked if I thought the surgery helped, I was shocked that the great success was not obvious. I was reborn at the age of 43. I stopped wearing pads and gradually rebuilt my life.

I know that the old doctor's tale of "it doesn't work" or "it won't last" is still being circulated, because when I suggest surgery to other women they report back that their doctor discouraged them from proceeding.

I am now 57. It has been 14 years since the surgery. I practice law in a small city and employ five people. I am a different person than that miserable, constantly depressed, withdrawn 43-year-old who had the surgery. I have no doubt that my life would be different in some ways if I had not spent ten years burdened as I was. Joey has always felt that I considered him a burden. I had wanted to have another child, but just never was up to it after his birth. I am fairly sure that had I received the help that I so diligently sought I would have returned to practicing law much sooner, or would have had another child.

The surgery I had did not become available when it did because it was a new development, it was simply denied to me earlier because the doctors I happened to see either did not know about it, or didn't approve of it.

Unfortunately I now weigh 250 pounds (so does Joey), but the surgery has held!!!!! At my current weight and age I can have a little incontinence and will wear a pad sometimes, but we are talking about drips not cups. For example, for a twelve-hour trip home from a cruise I wore a pad. I came home with no noticeable wetness. However, at 132 pounds and 32 years of age I could not walk to my car and drive for a half hour without being drenched in urine.

I have arthritis in my knees, no doubt aggravated by my weight, but if I was in a car accident and broke my leg no one would doubt that refusing to put a pin in my leg due to my weight would be anything other than heartless. Really, the traumatic delivery was the equivalent of an accident. It damaged my pelvic floor and made continence impossible.

I was injured bringing a child into the world – an intelligent and charming child who has grown into a loving husband and a responsible taxpayer. I deserved better treatment from the medical profession – and so did my family.

Resilience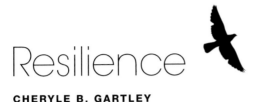

CHERYLE B. GARTLEY

EDITOR'S NOTE: For many individuals with incontinence, the loss of bladder or bowel control may be accompanied by other losses, including relationships, hobbies, or self-esteem. This can make it seem difficult to continue facing everyday life. This chapter examines what you can do to increase your own resilience so that you might return to a fuller, more hopeful life.

Defining Resilience

Resilience: 1) the capability of a strained body to recover its size and shape after deformation caused esp. [especially] by compressive stress. 2) an ability to recover from or adjust easily to misfortune or change.

Merriam-Webster's Seventh New Collegiate Dictionary

Simply put, resilience is the ability to bounce back from obstacles life throws in your path. This chapter is intended to help you better understand how life-challenges, including those unique to incontinence, can be lessened if you shape behaviors and build new skills that increase your resilience.

In *Resilience: Reflections on the Burdens and Gifts of Facing Life's Adversities,* author Elizabeth Edwards (the late wife of 2008 presidential candidate John Edwards) talks about the futility of wishing to have life as it was. "This is the life we have now, and the only way to find peace, the only way to be resilient when these landmines explode beneath your foundation, is first to accept that there is a new reality." The new reality for many people with incontinence is that while medical science continues to search diligently for a permanent solution to incontinence, the day-to-day challenges of living with a misbehaving bladder or bowel will cause stress.

We've all witnessed outstanding examples of resilience around us and wondered "Could I do that?" Whether we are observing a neighbor, a friend, or some stranger in the news, their resilience dazzles. Perhaps it's the Swedish fashion model whose boyfriend died in the tsunami, and yet she returns to that very place of heartbreak to build new schools; or it's the co-worker with cancer who returns to work the day after his treatments; or maybe it's the neighbor who lost a life-long job suddenly who leaves her house promptly each morning, day after day after day, to hunt for another position. Who are these people who can pick themselves up, dust themselves off, and carry on? Is it their faith, their life philosophy, a plain old attitude of the glass is half full – individuals who clearly say to themselves "If I can't change my life, I can change my attitude/behavior." And most importantly, how can we learn to be more like them when life knocks us down? Whether resilience is the word you use when you see these impressive people, you have in all likelihood seen the effects of resiliency in action.

Another way to think about resilience is as the ability to persist when things continue to go wrong. Calvin Coolidge (the 30th President of the United States) stated:

> Nothing in the world can take the place of persistence. Talent will not; nothing is more common than unsuccessful men with talent. Genius will not; unrewarded genius is almost a proverb. Education will not; the world is full of educated derelicts. Persistence and determination alone are omnipotent. The slogan 'Press On' has always solved and always will solve the problems of the human race.

Recognizing and Accepting Loss

Although we often use the phrase "loss of bladder and/or bowel control" in place of the word incontinence, we may not stop to recognize that indeed, for many, a substantial emotional loss has also entered their lives. Most people with incontinence have lost either part or all of their pre-incontinence lifestyles. They may no longer go sailing, play tennis, attend church, feel comfortable in a movie theater – all the "used to" activities that made up the fabric of their life seem less do-able. In fact, the term "social death" is sometimes used by experts when referring to the kind of social losses that accompany incontinence.

Author Susan Berger pointed out in *The Five Ways We Grieve* that everyone's grief is unique and the process happens in many ways. Although she is speaking about loss due to death, accepting incontinence and moving forward is also a process that requires:

- feeling the pain of loss,
- getting to the bottom of your feelings,
- finding ways to adjust to the new reality,
- contemplating the loss and exploring all the possible options now open to you for moving on.

Berger also comments that loss is "an experience that is final, life altering, and beyond your control … how you go on with your life and how you manage the impact of your loss, however, is very much within your control." It is important to note that by definition loss is beyond our control, which certainly applies to incontinence. It is also important to realize that loss, and the resulting (and often unrecognized) grief, can deprive us of hope.

One purpose of this chapter is to help reinstate hope in your life by giving you ideas on how to increase your resilience. Jerome Groopman writes eloquently about hope in *The Anatomy of Hope*, stating that "Hope can arrive only when you recognize that there are real options and that you have genuine choices." To have hope, then, is to acquire a belief in your own ability to have some control over your circumstances. As individuals experiencing incontinence, resilience can help us to focus on moving forward, finding options, and creating choices, so that we are no longer at the perceived mercy of forces outside of ourselves. Learning resilience skills can hasten the return of hope into our lives.

Victor Frankl, a psychiatrist who survived the concentration camps and later wrote *Man's Search for Meaning*, attributed the major difference between those who survived and those who did not, to hope: "As long as we are alive, humans are capable of forming images of what is possible, visualizing a better future, and creating a path to reach it." He wrote that the survivors were able to generate internal stamina that preserved them.

Resilience and Incontinence

Fortunately, more attention is now being paid to resilience, both within educational articles in the lay press and in academia, where researchers are beginning to study the skill-set needed to increase resilience. Scientists seem to agree that part of resilience is genetic and each of us is born with some level of inherent resiliency, but resilience, like any behavior, can also be learned.

It is not what happens to us that will have the greatest impact on our life, but rather how we think about what has happened, and how we respond. Philosopher Carl Buechner wrote, "People are disturbed not by things, but by the views which they take of them." Psychologists refer to changing our view of a life event as "reframing" the event. Lack of resiliency contributes to millions of people worldwide allowing their bladder and/or their bowel to take charge of their life. Learning to increase your resilience will help you wrestle control of your life (if not your bladder or bowel) back from these misbehaving muscles. You can "reframe" the impact of incontinence and live a life that is more of your own choosing.

The emotional response to leakage and its life impact is individual and not always correlated to the amount of urine or feces lost; so everyone needs a different reserve of resilience to bounce back. However, resilience is not something we are taught in school nor is it a skill often learned at home. Therefore many of us do not have a reserve of life skills we can apply to coping with a misbehaving bladder or bowel. Although studies show increased distress with certain types of leakage, it is common to see widely different life reactions to incontinence. One individual who manages leakage by wearing a small pad might be devastated. Yet, another person with total loss of control carries on quite well.

How Resilient Are You?

If this is the first time you've paid attention to the concept of resilience, then you might be wondering just how resilient you are. The following are some behaviors that indicate a lack of resilience, and others that show a good grasp of coping. Honestly assessing your own reactions to life's challenges is a good starting point.

Indications of lack of resiliency include:
- tending to dwell on problems rather than searching for solutions;
- feeling victimized;
- feeling overwhelmed;
- using unhealthy coping mechanisms such as abusing alcohol or sleeping pills.

Individuals who have developed resiliency are likely to have the following behaviors in their repertoire of coping skills:
- they stay connected with friends, family, and community;
- they attempt to find meaning in life;
- they examine what has helped in the past and then apply these same techniques to new challenges;
- instead of denying too long they make a plan and take action;
- they remain hopeful and make time to do enjoyable activities.

Additional characteristics of resilient people include: the ability to adjust their future expectations to fit their new reality; optimism; finding humor whenever possible; giving back when and where they can; spending time on what they can influence and not on the things they cannot control; and attempting to find the silver lining and gain strength from adversity. Resilient people do not view failures as end points and find no shame when they don't succeed. Instead they try to understand the reasons for a failure in order to use what they've learned to make the next attempt… to climb higher.

Wherever you feel you fall in the above lists of attitudes or skills, remember the habits that lead to poor resiliency can be broken, and the skills that lead to becoming a more resilient person can be increased.

You Can Increase Your Resilience

Resiliency is both a part of who we are (our individual personalities) and partly what we learn to do. Resilience can serve us in many ways – overcoming the obstacles of childhood, steering us through everyday adversities, helping us deal with major setbacks, and helping us achieve all we are capable of in life.

Obviously, increased resilience won't make life's problems go away. However, becoming more resilient can help us to enjoy life more, to look past the present difficulties, and hold onto hope for the future. It can help us to handle stress better. Achieving increased resiliency sounds like a tall order, especially around the challenges of incontinence, but taken in small steps, and by trusting in the process, you can learn some new skills that may help to change your life.

In their book *The Resilience Factor: 7 Keys to Finding Your Inner Strength and Overcoming Life's Hurdles*, authors Karen Reivich, PhD and Andrew Shatte, PhD speak about an individual's thinking style (the lens through which we view the world), because it colors the way we interpret the events in our lives. It is only human to assume that we are responding to an accurate picture of the world around us, when in fact our biases and thinking styles may be leading us to patterns of behavior that are often self-defeating.

> "Courage doesn't always roar. Sometimes courage is the quiet voice at the end of the day, saying, 'I will try again tomorrow.'"
> —Mary Anne Radmacher

Resiliency involves optimism, seeing problems or crises as challenges instead of curses, and avoiding regrets about the past. Optimism regarding incontinence might be associated with some of the following thoughts: scientists will solve this problem; new products and devices are coming to market; people like me for who I am, not for the state of my health; I can survive embarrassment because it is not the end of the world.

Resiliency involves flexibility and a solution orientation in problem solving. Coping is a dynamic process and having several strategies at hand is good.

Let the Work Begin

Creating the life you want takes work. Some of us learn this at an early age; for others this may be a news flash. Whichever category you fall into, most people will still find themselves at an impasse at some point when it comes to creating the life they want while living with a misbehaving bladder and/or bowel. Faced with an impasse, resilience can require a leap of faith, a willingness to act even before we believe that our actions will really improve our lives. There is no doubt that the longest mile begins with that first step.

Part of the issue of hopelessness may be the loss of comfortable life patterns we've developed, and the disconcerting ways they can be disrupted by incontinence. In his book *Getting Unstuck: How Dead Ends Become New Paths,* Dr. Timothy Butler refers to "patterns of the self." He suggests that for all of us, there are patterns to the things we like about the world, the things we value, the types of people and activities we tend to enjoy. Incontinence can temporarily interrupt many patterns in one's life from using your season tickets to the opera (front section center seats) to a weekend sailing in a boat that is too small to be equipped with a toilet. These interruptions come as a jolt. They disrupt our enjoyment of life and can plunge us into discouragement. But Dr. Butler writes that, in fact, without impasses in our lives we cannot grow, change, and eventually live more fully. "An impasse invites us to shed our fears and move to the border of what is actually presenting itself to us right now."

Feeling Stuck

If you feel stuck at an impasse due to your incontinence, taking even small steps to increase your resilience may be of help. Just the act of putting one foot in front of the other for a while can be amazing when you look back and see the distance you've traveled. The following are a few components of life, which when added together effectively, can alter your ability to bounce back.

Social Support: Millions of individuals are coping with their incontinence by giving up activities in order to stay close to a toilet. This behavior leads to losing contact with friends and family. If this sounds all too familiar, then one of the first steps to take is to commit to reversing this process. I'm not suggesting that you resume purchasing season tickets to the opera in a center seat where you'd be trapped until the curtain falls, but rather that you can find an activity which you'd enjoy and would bring people into your home and life on a regular basis – a book club, knitting circle (yes, real men knit), or simply inviting old friends over.

Thinking Styles: Most of us have never contemplated what our thinking style is, let alone tried to adjust it. So we are unaware that thinking styles can lead to patterns of behavior that are self-defeating. For instance, many people worry about events that have very little chance of actually happening. Others are not careful what they say to themselves, perhaps telling themselves that they should have found a way to solve their incontinence and haven't. All of us also have some fundamental beliefs of which we may not be aware. These beliefs may have served us well in other circumstances, but no longer do. Problem solving starts with accurate beliefs. Self-esteem starts with correct self-statements. Take time to examine your thinking style. It may lead you to the recognition that some changes would help build a better, more resilient outlook on life.

Optimism: Do you see problems as crises or as challenges? We aren't talking becoming Pollyanna (someone whose optimism is excessive to the point of naivete), nor in any way discounting the feelings that incontinence may cause, but rather it's about learning to have a perspective that allows you to say to yourself, "I'm faced with a challenge not a catastrophe." An action step to increase your resilience could simply be each time a problem (not just those related to incontinence) arises in your life, think about how you would rank the problem on a scale of one to ten. Also, examine your reaction; was it one of panic or of calm, collected thinking? Make a conscious effort to see your glass as half full, not half empty.

Avoid Hopelessness and Helplessness: Sometimes our life challenges mount up and there seems no escaping negative feelings like hopelessness. Accomplishing anything is often a start to vanquishing negative feelings – wash the car, clean out a long neglected closet, bathe your dog – in other words do something, then the next thing, and the next. Soon the process will help you to see that you are not helpless and you'll feel better.

Conclusion

Hopefully you were lucky and born with a wealth of innate resilience, but if not, remember that experts agree this is a skill that can be learned. Find a first step that suits you and then take it in order to move beyond the impasse that incontinence may be presenting in your life. Throughout this book, you will find many ideas, some of which will help you to grow, "press on," and create a more resilient life for yourself.

Further Reading

Harvard Business Review on Building Personal and Organizational Resilience. Boston: Harvard Business School, 2003.

Reivich, Karen, and Andrew Shatte. *The Resilience Factor: 7 Keys to Finding Your Inner Strength and Overcoming Life's Hurdles.* New York: Broadway Books, 2002.

Siebert, Al. *The Resiliency Advantage: Master Change, Thrive Under Pressure, and Bounce Back From Setbacks.* San Francisco: Berrett-Koehler, 2005.

Siebert, Al. *The Survivor Personality: Why Some People are Stronger, Smarter, and More Skillful at Handling Life's Difficulties... and How You Can Be, Too.* New York: Perigee Books, 1996.

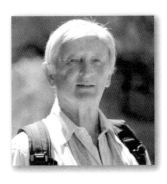

Incontinence as a New Element in My Life

WLODEK KOWALSKI, SWEDEN

EDITOR'S NOTE: This Lived Experience was originally written in Swedish. It has been translated into English.

Today is my birthday. One of many. Seven years have passed since I was told that I have cancer. The doctors suggested three half solutions: surgery, radiation, or waiting (see if the cancer manages to kill me before the day arrives for me to say goodbye to the world in another way).

We are not prepared for such situations. They surprise us and put our whole life on its head. The doctors do not tell you all the consequences. But even if they did that, we ourselves still have to make the final decision.

The first thought goes to what anyone with the barest knowledge of prostate cancer can expect, i.e. sexual potency in the future. I realized quickly that that business was finished. The decision I made was mine, only mine, and my wife accepted that decision.

The operation itself is only a question of whether to rely on or not rely on the surgeon. Since you don't have any choice, you have to rely on that person. You wake up after the trauma with a catheter installed and feel powerless, but not resigned. Hope remains; they will surely take the tube out, won't they?

No, it stayed there – for a long time – and when it was finally taken out, it turned out after several months that the cancer was not gone. In that situation, only radiation was left as the next move. To make a long story short, the consequence of the radiation left a fragile bladder and incontinence as a new element in my life.

The disappointment was big, despair grew over time. Irritation took over, and with it, the thought "why is this happening to me?" But after some time the situation became routine and an important and reassuring thought began – "why should it be unjust that this is happening to me?" Am I somehow better than others so that it should not strike me? If so, in what way and for what reason? And moreover, I – who have had so much good luck in my life and have a wonderful wife at my side, two wonderful sons, and two wonderful grandchildren – despite difficult years in my former homeland, had a worry-free childhood and younger years with a lot of love at home. Do I have the right to call what is happening to me now too unjust?

But it takes time to learn routines or rather to create them. "Hello, wake up, here is your new life that is talking – subject yourself to me, forget the old life!" To plan the days: "What errands do I have to do today, where is the nearest toilet, did I put an extra diaper in my pocket, do I have a plastic bag to throw away the package in? Do my clothes smell bad?" I do not notice it myself if I smell, think about something else...

I am the prisoner of my bladder, subject to its demands and unexpected whims, without control. It controls my life, my every day, my sleep, my drinking habits.

It started with the discovery that I drink too little water; the skin becomes drier, problems with discharge arise. That meeting with friends and having one or two beers wakes the alarm clock: "Go to the toilet before it is too late!" I am exiled for my handicap.

And then I come to an old political joke they told in communist Poland.

There is a party meeting in the factory. Everybody is forced to agree with everything being said, until a tractor driver gets up and asks for the floor.

Driver: Comrades, how can I meet my work quota if my tractor does not work?

Party secretary: Comrade, what is not working in it?

Driver: One wheel is broken.

Party secretary: Comrade, how many wheels does a tractor have?

Driver: Four.

Party secretary: Comrade, why this negative comment that focuses on a broken wheel instead of talking positively about the three that work well?

Yes! Why do I feel sorry about a part of my body that does not function as it should, instead of thinking about what fantastically well-functioning kidneys I have. They contribute certainly to my worries, but they function! And the rest of my body. I can sail, bike, work-out in the gym, go on hikes in the Greek mountains with my wife, work full-time despite my age, run after my beloved grandson who believes his grandfather cannot catch him, and go on vacations abroad.

A vacation abroad does, however, pose special challenges. A small suitcase must be packed with protective material for two weeks, mostly diapers, but also a urinal with associated tubes and bags, just in case. Also clean underwear for safety.

We land in Beijing after a cruise to Japan and South Korea, a two-week trip is just coming to an end and only the flight home is left. Then we are notified that no planes will fly today because of the Icelandic volcano, or rather its ashes. Panic!

After two days with a somber prognosis, our group of about 100 Swedish people gets together and discusses the problems that might come up shortly. Most people my age are worried about their medications running out. I tell them that I will soon not have any incontinence protection left.

And then that wonderful human quality makes its appearance: solidarity. Two men offer their protective diapers and a woman shares her medications. Such warmth.

Another trip: Leaving Egypt after a vacation stay. Nice memory, especially that the temperature was so pleasant that I perspired, sweating out part of the water which otherwise would have come out another way and would have become a problem near the pyramids where it is very hard to find a toilet.

But at the airport, a security person does not like the shape of my nose and after stupid questions about which religion I practice, he demands that I empty my pockets. I only have a spare diaper in my pocket. He picks it up with two fingers, and lifts it in the air and points scornfully at it for all passengers to see.

Surely, the incontinence restricts my life. Occasionally I am embarrassed. But thankfully the Swedish are a people who show a lot of tolerance and empathy, and that means that I do not have to be ashamed about my difficulties. And if you let go of the shame about your body, it suddenly becomes easier to live with incontinence or any other handicap whatsoever.

CHAPTER 9

Creating an Improved Quality of Life

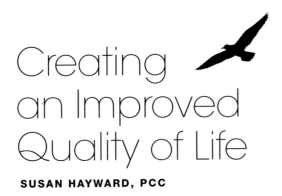

SUSAN HAYWARD, PCC

EDITOR'S NOTE: Living with incontinence may make you feel as though you've lost control of a large portion of your life. In this chapter Life Coach Susan Hayward will help you change the quality of your life, regain control of your choices and actions, and create new outcomes for yourself that are in line with your passions and values. By practicing the exercises included within the chapter you will have the opportunity to uncover specific and unique desires that you perhaps have put aside due to the impact of your incontinence.

Life is full of choices. You can choose to create the life you want, celebrate the life you already have in spite of your current upsets, challenges, and obstacles, and expand your vision beyond what you currently see for yourself (for instance, there is life beyond your misbehaving bladder or bowel). You are the best expert on you, and by creating your own answers to the questions in this chapter and by practicing the exercises, you will find you really do know what you want and that you can create it.

Application Is Always the Key

Application is always the key to change. You can read about change, learn about change, and talk about how to do it, but until you apply it to your life, nothing will change. The following life coaching strategies (modified from *Falling Awake* by Dave Ellis), with the exercises that are included, will guide you in applying new strategies to your own life.

Determining What You Want

Many of us wander through life without taking the time to really focus and decide on the life we would like to lead. As a life coach I help people create a specific, detailed vision for every area of their life, to identify short-term and long-term goals that are in line with their core values and passions. The objective of this chapter is to help you become more clear about your goals so that how you live your life is aligned with what you want.

As you uncover your desires for what you'd like your life to be, do not worry about how to accomplish them—that will come later. Create your vision by putting aside any doubt, all money concerns, fears regarding a misbehaving bladder or bowel, and current energy constraints. Let your passions guide you as you continue to ask yourself over and over, "What do I want?" For each answer to this question, then ask, "And what else do I want?" Keep moving and become more specific with each answer.

This process of getting more and more specific is very important. Think about how it would be if you went to eat at a restaurant, and you just ordered "dinner." You would have no idea what you might get and, more importantly, you would have no control over what you get. However, if you ordered baked pork chops, mashed potatoes with gravy, lettuce salad with French dressing on the side, steamed green beans, and unsweetened iced tea with lemon, that is exactly what you would get.

It is similar for the quality of life that you desire. You will get what you ask for. The purpose of identifying very specific desires and turning them into detailed goals is to capture a vision of the future you really want. As this vision becomes more and more clear, the vision itself will pull you forward into action.

It is important to determine your goals by creation, not prediction because of what has happened in the past. Prediction planning of goals keeps you stuck in the past and limits the possibilities for a new future. Creative planning of goals begins with a blank slate. Without considering the past, state what you want to have, do, and be in the present and future. From this detailed vision proceed to very specific goals—adding to those goals, timelines and possible partners for helping achieve your goals.

To begin Determining What You Want, use the exercises: *Wheel of Life* (see page 145) *and My Life Times Four* (see page 146).

Telling the Truth

It may be surprising to find out just how often you are not honest with yourself about what you _really want._ When you look closely at how you live your life, you may realize you have developed a habit of saying "I don't care" when asked by someone what you want, or saying "Whatever you want is fine with me," when it really isn't! How often have you been asked about what movie you want to go see and your response has been, "I don't care, you pick"? Yet when the other person picks a particular movie you immediately say, "Oh, but that movie didn't get a very good review. I want to see a five-star movie!"—so, you *did* really care.

Often you may not ask for what you want because you don't think the other person(s) will give it to you, therefore you accommodate your request to what you think they will give—or maybe you don't ask at all! Every time you do either of the above, you are giving away control over your life and letting someone else create your future for you. Denial about what you really want keeps you stuck where you are. Denying the truth about what you want takes a lot of energy and can result in chronic exhaustion or even illness.

Real honesty about what is working in your life and what you want to change is the beginning of the process of improving the quality of your life. Honesty allows everyone to become really clear about workable solutions to real obstacles in life.

Telling the truth is about speaking candidly, especially to yourself. How many times have you thought, "I should have said...," but you didn't because you were too frightened, too embarrassed, or too self-conscious to say it? When you stop yourself from speaking your truth, you cheat yourself out of the possibility of getting what you want. Refusing to speak your truth can cheat you and others of the opportunity to work on solutions together.

One way to practice telling the truth is to make and keep promises. You may like the word "agreements" or "commitments" instead of "promises." Substitute whatever word feels right as you read on.

Promises are reminders of what you want in your future; promises often become the goals that allow you to create your life experience. Promises can move you into action. Promises change intentions into reality. There are two ways to keep promises: one is to change your behavior so that it is consistent with your promises and the other is to change your promises so that they are in line with your behavior. When making promises, be sure they are "big enough" to challenge you into a desired action, but "not so big" that it is impossible to take the first step. Use promises to nudge yourself beyond your comfort zone. Big promises can be broken into a series of smaller promises such that each one prepares you for the next one—little by little. When your promises and behaviors are consistent with your core values, you experience a sense of control and a newfound freedom to create the life you want.

To practice Telling the Truth try the exercise *Talking to a Chair* (see page 147).

Taking Responsibility

Do you take responsibility for everything that happens in your life? This does not mean that you caused everything to happen. This does not mean you are to blame for everything that happens. What it does mean is that you are in control of your "response-ability" to all that happens in your life. Two very powerful questions can help shift your thinking to this new definition of responsibility:

1. "How did I create this?"
2. "How can I create a new result?"

To answer the first question, review the choices you made—or that you allowed others to make for you—that led up to the current situation in your life. Look at the consequences of those choices. You will often see that where you are or how you feel now is the direct result of something that you did or did not do (that you might have done) in your past. No one likes to admit that they actually contribute to some of the difficult circumstances in their life! Yet, it is precisely this admission that allows you to step out of the victim role and into the role of creating a new outcome by answering the second question above, "How can I create a new result?" You do not have to remain stuck where you are—especially in any situation you do not like. Your part in creating the situation may be a mere 10% or a huge 80%. The good news is that you are 100% in charge of your response to every situation.

> " *Your time is limited, so don't waste it living someone else's life. Don't be trapped by dogma – which is living with the results of other people's thinking. Don't let the noise of others' opinions drown out your own inner voice. And most important; have the courage to follow your heart and intuition. They somehow already know what you truly want to become. Everything else is secondary.* "
>
> —*Steve Jobs*

Perhaps one of your biggest fears is having an "accident" in public, because you are not 100% in control of your misbehaving bladder or bowel. As a result of this fear, you have isolated yourself in order to be absolutely sure this will never happen. Yet, when telling the truth to yourself you may find out how much you desire to participate more fully in life. By answering the question "How can I create a new result?" you can empower yourself to do something different and create several new possibilities for how to live your life.

One choice is to venture out in public every so often and hope to avoid an "accident" by "timing it right." Or you might choose to participate in the public arena often, knowing that the probability of having an "accident" is high. Acknowledging the reality of an "accident" allows you to then prepare ahead of time how you would like to respond when the "accident" happens. That preparation is another opportunity to explore many possibilities. As you continue to take responsibility for creating new results, you will create many possibilities for the life you want to live.

Another aspect of taking responsibility is to look at your interpretations of and assumptions about events in life. Whether aware of it or not, we are all interpreting life moment-to-moment. These interpretations create the degree to which we are happy and satisfied with our life. Begin paying attention to your interpretations of experiences. How many of those interpretations are based on assumptions, not on actual facts? It is often a habit to choose an interpretation (usually negative) based on an assumption (also usually negative) rather than to ask for clarity from others and actually get the facts before you respond to what someone else has "done" or "said." There are many interpretations for every experience in life. There is always the option of asking for clarity (the facts), or if that is not possible, choosing an interpretation that contributes to your happiness and well-being. Practice choosing interpretations that are both useful and accurate—interpretations that allow you to create your life the way you want it to be.

The following thoughts are possible examples of interpretations based upon an assumption that future experiences will be repeats of past experiences. For instance, do you often decline invitations to go out because you need to stop frequently to use the bathroom? You may have had a negative experience with someone in the past and therefore:

1. you are embarrassed to talk about your need,
2. you are afraid you might embarrass others by telling them of your need,
3. you believe that others will be inconvenienced by your needs, or
4. you believe others will become impatient with your need for frequent stops and become frustrated.

However, as you learn to ask for what you want, you can set the stage differently and actually ask how the other person feels about your concerns. For example, you might say, "I would love to go and I want you to know up front that I have a health issue that requires me to stop frequently to use the bathroom. To accommodate these numerous stops I want to plan for extra travel time. Does that work for you? Also, this problem often affects where I choose to sit so that I can easily exit with minimal disturbance to those around me. Do you know anything about the seating arrangements?"

Most people respond positively to direct requests and are relieved to know specifically what is expected and what they can do to be supportive. Vague and hesitant behavior often makes people ill at ease, because they want to help, but do not know how. Ask clearly and you will likely get what you want.

To practice Taking Responsibility use the exercises *Practice Taking Response-ability* (see page 148) and *Get the Facts* (see page 149).

Choosing and Managing Conversations

By expanding the definition of "conversation" and becoming aware of how to manage the many conversations in which you participate, the quality of your life will improve. The first image of conversation that most people have is of talking to and listening to another person. However, conversations also occur inside your head, especially when you struggle with any actions or behaviors that are not in alignment with your core values and beliefs. These conversations are usually critical, judgmental, full of "should haves," and greatly affect how we feel about ourselves. Additionally, we have conversations in our heads when reading a book, magazine article, or newspaper; watching television or listening to the radio; or even when we have dreams, daydreams, or nightmares.

At some level, although conscious of what we read, watch, and listen to, all of us are often unconscious of the conversations we internalize as thoughts and even beliefs, which then influence our mood, attitude, energy level, actions, and even self-esteem. To discover how these conversations affect you, begin by paying attention to how you feel after reading, listening to, or watching something of your choosing, or better still, when you are low on energy, in a bad mood, or feel out of sorts. Take a moment and think back to what you read, listened to, or watched in the past 24 – 48 hours. You may obtain insight into which conversations are influencing the way you feel. This information gives you the opportunity to experiment with changing your "conversations" or eliminating them altogether. You can usually choose who you spend time with, what you read, what you listen to on the radio, what movies you watch, and so forth. Pay attention to how you feel during and after your many "conversations," then become really clear about the conversations you want to keep as part of your life and those from which you want to walk away.

No matter which conversation you are in, it is important to balance your conversations. For instance, balance the tense (past, present, or future), the topics (things, other people, yourself), problems with solutions, and complaints with celebrations. Most of us have very strong conversation habits. Start by just observing the balance in your conversations. Then begin to look at balancing your conversations differently. If you find that you spend a lot of time talking about your problems, start spending more time talking about solutions to your problems. If you often talk about your worries for the future, spend more time talking about the realities of the present. You will immediately feel a shift in your attitude and energy level and feel more in control of the quality of your life.

It is very important to pay attention to the words you use. Words are very powerful— they create your consciousness and can determine attitudes as well as actions. These actions result in the circumstances of your life and create your unique and specific experience of life. In particular, pay attention to the words you use to describe your bodily functions. Do you use "leakage, incontinence, accident, urinate, flood, piddle, poop, bowel movement, etc." (add your own specific words to the list)? Read through this list of words slowly and pay attention to the feelings that each word creates in you. Do you feel embarrassed, demeaned, less than, disrespected? Do you feel differently when you use the word than when the same word is spoken by another person? Discover your comfort level with the words that you use to communicate with others and request that they use the same words. Choose words that empower, dignify, and value who you are beyond your bodily functions.

Finally, know that you can choose to enter conversations that align with your goals, desires and, interests and choose to leave those conversations that do not. Spend most of your time in conversations with people who support you in improving the quality of your life, affirm your goals and desires, and appreciate and celebrate who you are and what you want.

To practice Choosing and Managing Your Conversations follow the exercise *Tracking Your Conversation Habits* (see page 150).

Changing Habits

When changing a habit is mentioned, we usually think of New Year resolutions and the negative behaviors we want to stop. Instead, I encourage you to think about the positive habits you want to develop as a regular part of your life.

The first approach to changing habits triggers conversations in your head that lower your self-esteem and lead you to negative thoughts about yourself, your abilities, and your life. From this place, changing habits feels like lots of hard work.

The second approach to changing habits triggers those conversations filled with possibility, excitement, and anticipation of the improved quality of life you will have when you make a change. You feel encouraged and motivated to move to action. This action increases your self-esteem. You find strength in your abilities and you are empowered to improve the quality of your life without the drudgery of hard work.

For example, instead of saying, "I want to stop smoking," shift your thinking to, "I want to live a smoke-free life." The first approach feels like hard work and comes from a place of negative energy. The second approach is full of possibility and comes from a place of positive energy. Let me ask this question, "What if everything you do is just a habit?" I believe that if you adopt this position, then solving problems and getting what you want in life becomes as easy as taking charge of your habits. How often do you say, "I always…," "I never…,""That's just the way I am"? Take a moment to consider the possibility that your "always, never, and just how you are" are merely habits. It may really be just that simple! Remember that simple and easy are not synonymous.

Successfully changing habits involves awareness, commitment, tracking your progress, lots of practice, and celebration.

Before habits change, there must be an awareness of a desire for that change. This awareness includes getting very specific about how you want to change. Decide if you want to increase, decrease, eliminate, replace, or merely tweak a particular habit. Then quantify how much, how often, and by when.

Changing habits requires commitment. Once you are fully aware of the change you want, it is important to make a conscious commitment to that change, often in more than one way. You might write it down—in a diary, on an index card, or perhaps on a post-it note that you put in a place you will see daily. If you are on your computer a lot, make your commitment a screensaver! You might want to say it aloud to another person or to several people as a way to strengthen your commitment.

> " *Our lives improve only when we take chances … and the first and most difficult risk we can take is to be honest with ourselves.* "
> — *Walter Anderson*

Probably the most important step in changing habits is tracking your progress. Be sure to chart it, graph it, make tick marks in your calendar, or journal all of your successes. The tracking is your accountability system. If you have to write it down, you often think twice before repeating an old habit you want to change, and may instead eagerly practice new habits.

Lots of practice is involved in changing habits. Don't expect that just because you're aware of the change you want, you're committed to the change, and you have a great way to track it, the change will just happen! It won't. All change requires conscious and persistent practice. Accept that you might make a mistake sometimes. Acknowledge the mistake and re-commit to the change you want and practice some more.

Changing habits is not complete without celebration! It is important to celebrate small successes along the way. Every time you catch yourself practicing the change you want, celebrate. Create benchmark celebrations for consistency and persistence toward your desired change. And, of course, celebrate big when your change has been completely incorporated into your daily life. Here is an example that will walk you through the process you would follow in changing habits. You can substitute your own change as you read through this example.

Example: Perhaps you find yourself automatically saying no to any social invitation in an unfamiliar venue, because you're not sure if you can sit where you will be inconspicuous when you must "disappear" to the bathroom often to tend to your misbehaving bladder. A desired change might be to inquire about seating arrangements and bathroom locations before saying no to any social invitation in an unfamiliar venue. As you become aware of this desired change in habit, you determine that what you want to do is ask about seating arrangements and bathroom locations before saying no. This opens up the possibility of saying yes, and with that comes the anticipation and excitement about going out more often. You are now able to approach the change you want from a place of positive energy.

As part of making a conscious commitment, make several large reminders to post in significant places around your home and work environment—especially by the phone, your computer, and on a bathroom mirror. The notes simply say "ASK." On your computer screensaver you type in "Always ask before saying no!" Next you might tell your best friend about your commitment to ask. Sharing it with another person aloud always makes it more real and cements it in your consciousness.

Next you choose to make a graph where you record at the end of each day how many times you "asked" before deciding to accept or not accept a social invitation. You decide to track this for a minimum of three weeks.

Now you watch for opportunities to practice asking about seating arrangements and bathroom locations. If you slip up and say no too quickly, backtrack and say, "Oops, I forgot to ask. Before I say no, could you tell me about…?" And you practice asking over and over and over, until that is your new habit.

Deciding how to celebrate and how often is unique to each individual. Read more in the next section of this chapter and in the exercise titled *Ways to Celebrate*.

To practice Changing Habits follow the steps outlined in *5 Steps to Changing a Habit* (see page 151).

Learning to Celebrate

Celebration is about shifting the focus of your energy from the negative to the positive. Celebration is about nurturing yourself and declaring that your life deserves to be celebrated. Celebration is meant to help you recognize that even in the midst of the chaos and turmoil that at times seems to dominate your life, there are things that are positive and for which you are grateful. Another way to say it is that even when some things are not working well, there are always some things that are working well, which deserve your acknowledgement and celebration. For example, in the midst of dealing with a misbehaving bladder or bowel, you still might celebrate your successes at work, the love of your family, the support of a medical professional, a good book you read, the laugh of a child, the safety of travel, or the joy of listening to music. The list might be quite long and will put into perspective the distress of dealing with your misbehaving bladder or bowel.

Along the way to changing your habit, plan some benchmark celebrations that motivate you to keep practicing until the change in habit is complete. A benchmark celebration for me might be meeting a friend for coffee and a snack at a coffee shop. The final celebration—when your habit is a consistent part of your life—should be something that you really look forward to having or doing. A final celebration for me would be taking a day of rest and relaxation during the week at a nearby state park. However you choose to celebrate, enjoy it fully!

With practice, celebration empowers you with positive energy to take charge of your life and create what you want in spite of any chaos or turmoil present at the moment. Engaging in regular celebration builds a strong foundation for seeing that the other side of a complaint can be an opportunity for change, and that obstacles can be opportunities for personal growth. Celebration allows you to affirm the positive in the midst of the negative. When turmoil and chaos bring negative energy into your life, celebration allows the positive energy already present in your life to break through that negativity. Celebration is a reminder that you have a choice every moment to be upset or to be happy, to be proactive, or to be the victim of your circumstances. Celebration helps you move into the positive choices.

As you become more aware of everything that is going well in your life and take time to celebrate it, you actually begin to see more and more of what is working well in the midst of life circumstances that are not as you wish them to be. Celebrating empowers you to take charge of your life and create what you want rather than reacting to whatever comes your way. In celebration is the recognition of the hope you have through the power of seeing possibility. And as you act on those possibilities you begin to take charge of the changes you want in your life.

To learn how you like to celebrate, apply ideas from the exercise *Ways to Celebrate* (see page 152).

Choose to Take Action

The truth is, you are the only expert on you. You are the one who knows what you really want. By paying attention to what you want—not what others want, nor what you think you should want—you can make new choices that move you into actions that create the life you want to live. It is never too late to listen to yourself and choose to ask for what you want, do what you really want to do, and be who you really are.

Some important questions are: How committed am I to moving away from the stuck places in my life? Am I willing to look beyond my complaints to the desires they over-shadow? Am I willing to find the possibilities hidden in the obstacles before me? Do I want to move away from the familiar to discover new possibilities?

Many of the ideas within this chapter have come from my training and experience as a life coach. If change doesn't come easily for you or you get stuck for too long, you might want to consider getting some focused help from a professional trained as a clinical social worker, a psychologist, a psychiatrist, or a life coach. By interviewing various professionals you are likely to find a good fit, whether you want help sorting out a tangle of problems, clarifying what it is you do want, or coaching you through the process of changing patterns of thinking and behavior. Ask professionals to describe how they work with clients like you. Do the approaches they describe seem like a good fit for your concerns and personality?

I encourage you to begin by trying the exercises offered at the end of this chapter to empower yourself and to enhance the quality of your life. You are worth the time and effort!

Wheel of Life

(Determining What You Want)

Directions: The eight sections in the **Wheel of Life** represent various parts of life.

1. Rank your level of satisfaction in each life area by filling in a curved arc in each section. The center point is zero (very dissatisfied) and the outer arc is ten (very satisfied).

2. Identify three changes that would improve your level of satisfaction within each area of your life as it is today. These can be short-term or long-term changes. List the changes briefly near each section of the wheel.

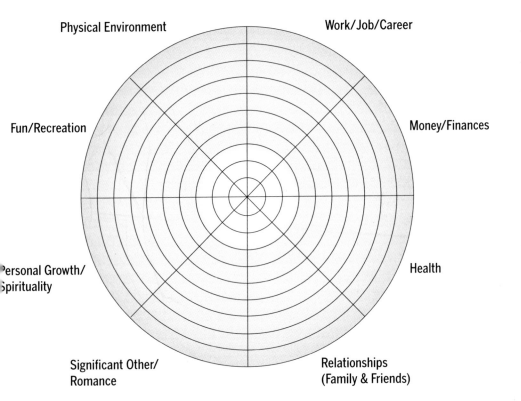

My Life Times Four
(Determining What You Want)

Create a new vision of your future by identifying goals that would double the satisfaction of your current life situation. Now, take that vision and create goals to double your satisfaction with that vision.

When you fill out the details of your vision, you will often find that not everything shows up exactly the way you envisioned it. However, the more specific you are about what you want, the more easily you can recognize it when it comes in a slightly different form from your original imagining.

With this visioning exercise, it is not necessary to know how to achieve your goals—just remain open to the sense of possibility of what you want.

Experiment with capturing your vision/goals in various media—writing, drawing, sculpting, painting, making a collage, recording yourself as you speak aloud.

Have fun!

Talking to a Chair
(Telling the Truth)

Place an empty chair in front of you. Sit in another chair so that you are facing the empty chair. Decide who you would like to sit in the empty chair so you can tell them a truth you have been withholding. You might ask, "Who should I place in that chair?" I suggest it be someone you are upset with, someone you are afraid of, someone who has hurt you, someone who has abandoned you, or someone you care about deeply.

Once you have put that other person in the chair in your imagination, begin speaking aloud to them as if they were actually sitting in your presence. Address them by name and tell them the truth you have been withholding.

You will become empowered by speaking aloud the truth, even when the person you are talking to is not physically present.

This practice may be the first step towards being able to actually tell the truth to the other person face to face, on the phone, or in a letter.

Practice Taking Response-ability
(Taking Responsibility)

The three steps of this problem solving exercise are Describe a Problem, Determine Your Role, and Decide on a Solution.

Describe a Problem: Pick one problem in your life that you would like to resolve. Describe it in detail. Describe how it will be when the problem is resolved.

Determine Your Role: List all the possible ways that you are keeping the problem from being resolved. Take responsibility for your role(s) in continuing the problem by telling the truth in an objective, nonjudgmental way. The purpose of this exercise is to discover the behaviors that you can change to bring resolution to the problem.

Decide on a Solution: Review the description of your problem, the description of the problem resolved, and the list of ways you are keeping the problem from being resolved. Pick one specific behavior from your list and state how you intend to change this behavior. Be specific about how this change in behavior will help solve the problem. Practice this new behavior for a predetermined length of time to see if it solves the problem. If not, go back to the list and select another behavior and repeat the process. Sometimes a change in behavior may lessen the problem, but not solve it completely. In this case, you will want to continue that behavior change while also changing another behavior from your list in order to completely solve the problem.

If you want to tackle more than one problem at a time, go through this exercise separately for each problem you want to resolve.

Get the Facts
(Taking Responsibility)

Facts come from observable actions. Everyone witnessing the same actions will report the same facts *and* possibly different interpretations. Interpretations are about the meaning of a specific action. Interpretations cannot be directly observed. Interpretations come from each person's past experience with and understanding of the observed action. We often react to our interpretations of an action rather than first determining the facts. This often further complicates the situation.

To determine the difference between the facts and your interpretations for any circumstance, do the following:

■ Select a specific circumstance that has upset you.

■ Make a list of the facts that you observed.

■ Review the list to see how many of your facts really are interpretations.

As you practice picking out facts from interpretations you will shift from reacting in nonproductive ways to responding responsibly. You will gain clarity about an appropriate response you want to take and you will decrease the distress that often comes from reacting to interpretations rather than taking the time to get the facts.

Tracking Your Conversation Habits

(Choosing and Managing Your Conversations)

For a specified length of time, commit to paying attention to your conversation habits. It could be a day or two or even up to a week. Remember that conversations are not just interactions with others—they also include what you think, listen to, and read.

Focus on one habit at a time: tense, topic, circumstances, or attitudes. The order is not important. You might begin by consciously focusing your awareness on the tense of your conversations. Do you spend most of your conversation time talking, thinking, listening to, or reading about the past, the present, or the future? In the chart below, estimate the percent of time you spend in each tense. Repeat this intentional focus with each of the other conversation habits.

Conversations:			
Tense	Past _____%	Present _____%	Future _____%
Topics	Things, Events, or Other people _____%	You _____%	Me _____%	Us _____%
Circumstances	Problems, Issues, or Concerns _____%	Solutions _____%		
Attitude	Complaints _____%	Celebrations _____%		

After tracking your conversations, review the above chart to identify your conversation habits. You may choose to write intentional goals for any changes you want to make in managing your conversation habits. For example, your tracking may have indicated that you spent 80% of your conversation time on problems and only 20% of your time on solutions. An intentional goal might be "I intend to spend 40% of my conversation time on my problems and 60% on creating solutions."

5 Steps to Changing a Habit
(Changing Your Habits)

1. **Become aware** of the habit you want to change and determine exactly how you want to change it. (Eliminate it, replace it, or tweak it.)

2. **Make a commitment** to change the habit. (Write it down in your diary, write it on an index card, or tell someone else about your commitment.)

3. Decide how to **track your progress.** (Chart it, graph it, make tick marks on a 3 X 5 card, track it in your calendar, or journal about it.)

4. **Practice, practice, and practice** the change in habit. (Practice without reproach and with persistence.)

5. **Celebrate** all your successes in changing the habit. (Celebrate benchmarks along the way, reward yourself for progress as it happens. Do not wait until the habit is completely changed to celebrate, especially if it is a big/difficult habit to change.)

Ways to Celebrate
(Learning to Celebrate)

The words "celebrate" and "celebration" may conjure up images that just don't fit into your current life experience. You may want to substitute another word like "grateful/gratitude," "blessings," "wins," or "accomplishments." Use whatever word resonates with you. Perhaps with time you will find that "celebration" becomes an important part of your daily life. Celebrations can be small or huge, personal or universal, about yourself (your health, finances, job/career, spirituality, physical environment, etc.), about your interactions with others, about others who are important in your life, or about whatever else you consider a celebration.

Below are suggestions for beginning a celebration practice. Choose whichever ones speak to you—or better yet, create your own style of celebration.

1. Write down a list of your celebrations daily. Writing them down is important.

2. Write about your celebrations in your diary. Elaborate on the details of the celebration, its impact on your life, or how you feel about a particular celebration.

3. Create a card file of celebrations by category and watch the various sections grow with time and as you become more aware of all you have to celebrate.

4. Find a celebration partner with whom to communicate regularly. Email is a great way to share celebrations with someone else, as are phone conversations.

5. Create a space and ritual for celebrating. Designate a particular place in your home where you go to celebrate. Light a candle, put on your favorite music, and practice deep breathing before capturing your celebrations.

6. Make a collage of significant celebrations and place it where you can see it often.

7. Organize a basket of things you like to do that you don't often take the time to do. My basket has a scented candle, a favorite CD, a set of juggling balls, a book of poetry, and a deck of cards.

8. Treat yourself to something special. Enjoy a favorite beverage at a local coffee shop, visit a local museum, eat lunch at your favorite restaurant, by yourself or with a friend.

9. Buy something for yourself that is relevant to what you are celebrating. For example, someone who was working on managing her conversations by successfully walking away from non-productive conversations decided to buy herself a new pair of shoes to celebrate her success.

However you choose to celebrate is up to you. The desired outcomes of celebrations are that you complete your celebration time in a positive mood, you feel refreshed and relaxed, and are re-energized.

Life with Incontinence

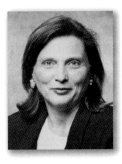

NANCY J. NORTON, USA

I have lived with bowel incontinence for 24 years as the result of an obstetrical injury. I have told my story many times as the Founder of the International Foundation for Functional Gastrointestinal Disorders. A moment in time changed the course and path of my life in ways I never could have imagined. I have been blessed and honored to achieve many things in life that I would have never accomplished if I had not become incontinent. Building a patient organization was not in my plans or thoughts before this happened to me.

In my previous life, as I think of it, I was a textile artist and conservator. I still have a great appreciation for textiles from all cultures, enjoying ethnographic art and all that it has to reveal. I still view myself as an artist, but for the past twenty years my focus has been quite different. I have worked to raise awareness about functional gastrointestinal and motility disorders and the need to increase research to find better treatments, and ultimately cures, for people like myself.

Having said all of this, reliving the medical details of the birth experience and what followed, which redirected my life, is like pouring salt on an open wound. The passage of time has not made it easier. I had two unsuccessful repair surgeries that were hideously painful and debilitating. I sought help from some of the best medical institutions in the U.S. at the time, and attempts were made to help me. In the end I was left with the words, "You will just need to learn to live with this." But no one could tell me how to even begin to learn to live with incontinence, a bowel disorder that left me fearful of leaving home. I felt lost. As I was a new mother struggling to recover from multiple surgeries, my husband was always there for me and our son. With his help and support I slowly was able to find my way forward.

It took time to sort through the disbelief, anger, and sorrow that followed. A sense of loss remains ever present. The future that once seemed so clear was now veiled with uncertainty. Choices had to be made. The path that I chose was one of not feeling that I needed to hide my incontinence. I had already seen too much of that in life. My mother had been totally disabled by multiple sclerosis (MS) and had lost both bladder and bowel function.

She was unable to care for herself and was reliant on others. I remember her saying as tears filled her eyes that she "needed to maintain her dignity." As a young child I had no idea of the depth of her words, but I could see how painful the experience was for her. Clearly, at that time the ravages and realities that accompany diseases were seldom discussed. No one wanted to know about bowel and bladder problems. People could talk about MS, but no one talked about everything that accompanies it. When unavoidable, that discussion was whispered behind closed doors.

Decades later, when I became incontinent, it seemed little had changed. Many people did not want to hear about how my life had changed and the difficulties I experienced. Some friends and acquaintances slipped away; but other people stood by my husband and me and remain close friends.

Feelings of hopelessness filled me for several years after I became incontinent. I never would have believed then that I would have a future doing the things that I have since been able to do. I became afraid to leave my home for fear of being incontinent in public, and the feelings of embarrassment and shame that accompany that. The shame and stigma associated with incontinence are deeply rooted in cultural norms; despite the public role that I have developed, I never cease to feel them.

After I became incontinent, there no longer was spontaneity in my life. I felt as if I was ruled by the incontinence. Just getting to my local physician was a challenge. Traveling half-way across the country to see a specialist seemed next to impossible. With nothing to guide me, I had to figure out how to start getting a handle on this. I needed to overcome the uncertainty around being incontinent, or at least learn how to minimize it, if I was going to be able to get back into the world. So I began with learning how to manage this condition. It was small steps to begin with.

I had been to college and graduate school, and thought that maybe it would be a good idea to try to take a class at the local university. I thought of it as something that would get me out of the house. I would have to sit in a room with other people for an hour and try not to let my anxiety get the better of me. I took a class on public policy to learn about advocacy. Making sure to know where the restroom was located and being prepared in the event that I lost continence, I was able to get to the classes and complete the course. This first step gave me a little more confidence to keep going.

I am a person who likes to see tangible and positive results for things I take on, but my incontinence has not improved over time, so that tangible change did not occur for me in the way I had hoped. Instead I had to look at changing how I thought and operated in the world, which was no easy task. I have learned to live with being incontinent, essentially with the help for many years of a biofeedback therapist. I am always watchful of what and when I eat, take anti-diarrheal medication, especially when traveling or when I need to be out of my office for the day, and make sure I get enough sleep. Thinking about maintaining the consistency of stool in order to prevent losing it is a 24-hour, seven-days-a-week challenge for me. I am always prepared with clean-up supplies and basically still take each day one at a time.

I have worked for many years to help diminish the stigma around incontinence, but it continues to be a challenge. Marketing messages encourage us to buy products to hide this condition from everyone, even friends. Society perpetuates the notion that incontinence is something not to talk about. Few people even tell their doctors, and data shows that less than one in four physicians will ask their patients about loss of bladder or bowel control. The reference to "adult diapers" conveys a message that goes far beyond the words, one that carries an infantile connotation that diminishes a person. It may seem insignificant to some, but I believe that it continues to feed a message that makes it even more difficult to reveal symptoms of incontinence.

After 24 years of living with incontinence I know what the challenges are. I know how difficult it is to carry on, and to find a way to function and fit into society. I wish I could say that the medical community as a whole has made progress in this area, but unfortunately there continue to be few options to help people like me. I have spoken with thousands of people over the years who live with and feel the same frustration. We have made some progress with awareness, but we remain a long way from being a culture in which people who suffer incontinence can feel comfortable revealing their symptoms and struggles.

Still, I remain optimistic. I know there are clinicians and researchers who are searching for improved treatment methods. There are people in industry that are trying to understand the needs and concerns of people with incontinence, and how best to address them. I know there are advocates who work on behalf of all of us. I only wish there were more.

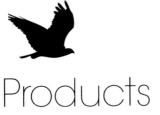

CHAPTER 10

Products and Practical Management

CHRISTINE NORTON, PhD, RN

EDITOR'S NOTE: When first facing incontinence, many people will find something—anything—that helps deal with the problem. Once you find something that stops or conceals the leakage, it isn't uncommon to stop looking for further solutions. However, it's possible that there are better options out there. This chapter will present many of the products that are now available, along with guidance as to what you can realistically expect from those products. Additionally, helpful tips are provided for steps that you can take to more effectively manage your incontinence.

Using the best possible products can make a big difference to your life with incontinence. It is important to try different products to find out which ones you will find the most secure and comfortable. Different criteria are important to each of us, so you can decide what your priorities are:

- Comfort
- Security from leakage
- Odor control
- Does not rustle or make a noise
- Easy to use
- Easy to carry both daily and in bulk when travelling
- Easy and discreet to dispose of when used
- Does not show under clothes

Few products are perfect, so you may have to accept a trade-off between some of your criteria. For example, bigger diapers are likely to be more absorbent (but not always so), but less easy to hide under clothes or dispose of in rest rooms.

New products are being developed all the time, so it is worth checking from time to time that nothing better has come along. Visit www.continencecentral.org for a list of sources of information on products. Because products change so often, this chapter will not talk about specific brands or companies, but will describe general types of product. But be aware that within each type there are many brands of varying quality, and quality or performance does not always relate directly to price (more expensive is not necessarily better!). It is difficult to predict how an individual product will work for each person, and there really is no way to tell except trying it.

Products for Managing Urinary Incontinence

Pads, Pants, and Diapers

Some people adamantly refuse to wear pads because they view this as a sign that they "have given in" and therefore have to accept their symptoms. Others use very large pads or diapers "just in case," even though episodes of incontinence are actually very rare.

The simplest pad for minor leakage is a panty liner, available in supermarkets and drug stores. However, this will not cope with more than a few drops of urine.

For individuals who have leakage that occurs infrequently, it may be reassuring to wear washable pants with a built-in waterproof gusset, especially if you will be away from the toilet for a long period of time. These should stop any leaks from getting through to your clothes.

More major incontinence will require larger pads. These come in many shapes and sizes, including rectangular or shaped inserts, all-in-one diaper-style, and T-shaped pads with a waist belt. Different pads of the same size may have very different absorbencies, depending on the design and quality of the materials used. Products that work well when you are standing may work less well when you are sitting or lying on your side. For men there are "leaf-shaped" pads that fit over the penis and scrotum.

There is also a large variety of bed pads, mattress protectors, and pillow and duvet covers. Some are washable, others are disposable. More expensive bedding protection may be made of a "breathable" fabric which can feel less hot.

Penile Sheaths (Condom Catheters)

These are suitable for men with urinary incontinence. An adhesive sleeve is rolled over the penis. This is usually connected to a leg bag by day and may be connected to a larger urine collection bedside bag at night. Sheaths should be used with care because skin damage can result if they are applied too tightly, the adhesive is pulled off too roughly, or if the skin is not cared for by washing, drying, and allowing some time without the sheath.

Catheters

A catheter is a small, hollow tube inserted into the bladder to drain out urine. There are three main types:

- An **intermittent catheter** is one that you insert via the urethra (bladder outlet) several times a day if your bladder does not empty very effectively. Draining out the urine that is sitting in your bladder (residual urine) can keep you dry between catheterisations and may also help to prevent urinary tract infections. Many people can use intermittent self-catheterisation (ISC) by learning to insert a catheter several times each day. Others will need a caregiver to help with this. Many can learn to use ISC sitting on almost any toilet.

- An **indwelling urethral catheter** (often called a Foley catheter) stays in the bladder all the time and may be connected to a leg bag or an overnight bag, or have a catheter valve attached, which you can release over the toilet every few hours. There is a small balloon attached that is inflated inside the bladder to keep the catheter in place. The catheter is usually changed every few months. Though not without its own problems, an indwelling catheter will keep some people with heavy incontinence dry.

- A **suprapubic catheter** is similar to an indwelling catheter, but is inserted into the bladder via a small hole (made under local anaesthetic) in the lower abdominal wall. This can be connected to the same bags or valves as for urethral catheters.

The decision to use a catheter will be one for you to discuss with your health care practitioner, who will need to monitor your kidney function from time to time.

Products for Managing Fecal Incontinence

There are no perfect answers to the problem of coping with leakage from the bowel. It is very difficult to find anything that reliably disguises bowel leakage and odor, and very few products have been designed specifically for fecal leakage.

Anal Plugs

Some people with minor leakage of mucus or stool from the anus find that a small piece of cotton or cotton wool, rolled between the fingers and then gently inserted just inside the anus, with the use of lubricant to aid insertion if required, will stop the problem.

A specially designed anal plug has been developed. It comes wrapped up in a water-soluble film and should be covered with lubricant so that it is easy to insert. The film dissolves once inside the rectum, and the plug opens into a cup shape, with a string for removal from the anus. It comes in two sizes, small and large. It can be left in place for up to 12 hours and removed by pulling on the attached cord.

This is a useful device for people who leak stool from the bowel without any feeling (passive soiling). You can use it on a daily basis or when you do sports activities. It is not really suitable for people with a high bowel frequency because it would need to be removed each time. The advantage of this device is that it usually stops soiling. However, many people find it uncomfortable to wear, and the majority cannot tolerate it. For this reason it is most suitable for people with neurological conditions, such as a spinal injury or spina bifida, because they frequently lack good sensation in the anal canal.

The plug cannot be flushed down the toilet, and so must be wrapped in paper or a disposal bag and put in the rubbish bin.

Pads, Pants, and Diapers

There are very few pads designed specifically for managing fecal incontinence. Most of the disposable pads used for urinary incontinence can be used for containment, but some patients find them unnecessarily thick, bulky, and not the right shape or length to contain soiling from the anal canal.

Unfortunately, if pads are used inside pants, the area around the anus often becomes sore as the stool leaks onto the skin initially before reaching the pad. Some patients have found that folding a panty liner between the buttocks and holding it in place with a close-fitting "G-string" helps to contain soiling and prevent soreness or excoriation. Some panty liners have a soft cover, which seems to be softer than a "stay dry" cover.

> "What I know for sure is that your life is a multipart series of all your experiences — and each experience is created by your thoughts, intentions, and actions to teach you what you need to know. Your life is a journey of learning to love yourself first and then extending that love to others in every encounter. The big secret in life is that there is no big secret. Whatever your goal, you can get there if you're willing to work."
> —Oprah Winfrey

Adapting the Bathroom

If you have any type of disability, you may find that adaptations to your bathroom make life with incontinence easier. This might include installing some rails to make sitting on the toilet feel more secure, or to assist in sitting down and getting up again. There are also raised seats if your hips do not bend easily and even spring-loaded seats to help you stand up from the toilet. If you use a walker or wheelchair, you may need to think about bathroom re-design to make transfer easy.

Using an Alternative to the Toilet

If getting to or onto the toilet is impossible, there is a variety of disposable or washable products that can be used for urination or defecation. Some are simple camping devices or portable potties designed for children who are not yet fully trained. Others are more permanent devices such as a commode chair or a washable urinal. A specially designed cone is available that allows women to urinate while standing up for those who cannot sit easily or need to urinate in a hurry without removing clothing (maybe on a country walk behind a bush).

Washing and Odors

Many people who experience incontinence frequently plan their journeys by "toilet stops" (sometimes referred to as toilet mapping). This helps to alleviate some of the anxiety, but if the bladder or bowel is unpredictable, incontinence can still occur. Carrying a "spares kit" to enable clean-up and a change of clothes can give added confidence, and for some this acts as a security blanket—less anxiety may make accidents less likely.

Public restrooms seldom have a washbasin in the cubicle, and trying to get clean with dry toilet tissue is difficult and can be painful for those with sore or excoriated skin. Therefore, wet wipes are preferable to remove all traces of urine or feces. Alternatively, carry a small plastic bottle that can be filled with warm water to take into the cubicle and used to wash. Clothes pegs are useful to keep clean clothes out of the way, particularly if you are not very nimble with your fingers. The pegs can be used to hold up skirts or shirts and prevent dangling onto soiled areas or the toilet bowl. A small pocket mirror is useful for checking that the perineal area is clean and that there are no apparent stains on clothing before leaving the restroom.

There are many different sanitary towel or nappy sacks (disposable diaper bags) for sale, which are useful for disposal of pads or to carry home soiled clothes. Many are slightly scented, which helps to disguise the smell of the contents. Odors from urine, gas, or stool can be disguised by a small neutraliser or spray perfume if you are concerned. If you buy these online or at a pharmacy, the deodorants designed for people with an ostomy are most suitable.

Skin Care

Anyone who has urinary or bowel incontinence or frequent bowel movements may get sore skin from time to time. This can be very uncomfortable and distressing. Occasionally, the skin may become so inflamed that it breaks into open sores. These are then difficult to heal. Taking good care of the skin can help to prevent these problems from developing.

The skin can become sore due to a variety of reasons. Constant moistness leads to irritation. Chemicals contained in the bacteria of stool and digestive enzymes are skin irritants. Diarrhea is likely to contain a higher content of digestive enzymes because there has been less time for the colon to re-absorb these. The presence of both urinary and fecal incontinence together seems to exacerbate the tendency to soreness. Frequency of defecation leads to repeated wiping, which can damage the sensitive skin of the anus.

Wiping with dry paper seems to be more traumatic than using a wet wipe.

Some anal conditions such as haemorrhoids make it very difficult to wipe effectively. Any stool remaining after wiping causes irritation, and scratching the area causes soreness.

If you are not eating a healthy balanced diet, not drinking enough, or not taking much exercise you are more prone to soreness, as well as if you are generally unwell and not very active or mobile.

Tips to Prevent Soreness

With careful personal hygiene it is often possible to prevent soreness, even if you have incontinence.

- Always use soft toilet paper GENTLY, or ideally the newer moist toilet paper (available from larger pharmacies and some supermarkets). Discard each piece of paper after one wipe, so that you are not re-contaminating the area you have just wiped.

- Whenever possible, wash after you have been incontinent. A bidet is ideal (portable versions are available). If this is not possible, you may be able to use a shower attachment with your bottom over the edge of the bath. Or use a soft disposable cloth with warm water. Avoid washcloths and sponges, because they can be rough and are difficult to keep clean. Sometimes a little ingenuity is needed, especially if you are away from home. Some people find that a small plant sprayer, watering can, or jug filled with warm water makes washing easy on the toilet or over the edge of the bath.

- Do not be tempted to use disinfectants or antiseptics in the washing water because these can sting, and many people are sensitive to the chemicals in them. Just plain warm water is best.

- AVOID using products with a strong perfume, such as scented soap, talcum powder, or deodorants, on your bottom. Choose a simple nonscented soap (e.g., a baby soap). Many baby wipes contain alcohol and are best avoided.

- When drying the area BE VERY GENTLE. Pat gently with soft toilet paper or a soft towel. Do not rub. Treat the whole area as you would a newborn baby's skin. If you are very sore, a hairdryer on a low setting may be most comfortable (use carefully!).

- Wear cotton underwear to allow the skin to breathe. Avoid tight jeans and other clothes that might rub the area. Women are usually best to avoid tights and to use stockings or crotchless tights instead. Use nonbiological washing powder for underwear and towels.

- Avoid using any creams or lotions on the area, unless advised to do so. A few people who are prone to sore skin do find that regular use of a cream helps to prevent this. If you do use a barrier cream, choose a simple one (such as zinc and castor oil), use just a small amount, and gently rub it in. Large amounts stop the skin from breathing and can make the area sweaty and uncomfortable. Make sure that the old layer of cream is washed off before applying more. Some people are allergic to lanolin, and creams containing this should be avoided.

- Your doctor or nurse may suggest using a barrier wipe which forms a protective film over the skin, especially if you have diarrhea and are opening your bowels very frequently.

- If you need to wear a pad because of incontinence, try to make sure that no plastic comes into contact with your skin and that you use a pad with a soft surface.

- Whenever possible, unless you have been advised not to for other reasons, eat a healthy, balanced diet, drink plenty of water, and take as much exercise as you can. Some people find that certain food or drink makes them more prone to soreness, especially citrus fruit such as oranges. It may be worth cutting these out on a trial basis, and more permanently if this helps.

Note: Women are advised always to wipe front to back (i.e. AWAY from the bladder and vaginal openings) because bacteria from the bowel can infect the bladder and vagina if you wipe from back to front.

If you are already sore, you are advised to follow all of the advice above on prevention. In addition, damp cotton wool may be found to be the most comfortable to use for wiping. A simple barrier cream or ointment may be enough to allow the skin to heal. If drying the skin after washing is difficult or uncomfortable, a hairdryer on a low setting may be used, but with great care. Try not to scratch the area, however much you are tempted, as this will make things worse. If you find that you scratch during sleep at night, wearing cotton gloves in bed (available from a drugstore/chemist—more usually used for people with skin conditions such as eczema) may help. It is important to allow air to get to the sore area for at least part of every day.

An Unpleasant Condition

TZIPI, ISRAEL

EDITOR'S NOTE: This Lived Experience was originally written in Hebrew. It has been translated into English.

I am 64, married, and the mother of three children who were born by vaginal delivery. I worked as a hospital nurse for around thirty years, and then I felt the need to do something completely different. I have spent the past 14 years designing and manufacturing costumes for the theater and for dance troupes. I have found satisfaction in my diverse work.

I don't remember when I began to "suffer" from urinary incontinence, since it didn't happen overnight, but I can recall a few episodes of incontinence when I laughed heartily. You know what people say: "I laughed so hard I peed in my pants," and I wasn't especially concerned.

But as time went by, and this was around twenty years ago, I noticed that these were not isolated episodes, and that it didn't happen only when I laughed. It also happened when I was engaged in various other activities. For instance, we were members of a fitness club that we went to around three times a week. When I was on the treadmill and the speed was pretty high, I would have episodes of urinary incontinence. I would have to go to the bathroom and change my pants, despite the absorbent pads that I used. That was also why I made sure to wear only black pants—the only color I allow myself to wear. But that wasn't such a big deal either.

The urinary incontinence became more severe and happened on other occasions too, such as our regular monthly hikes with a group. It happened mainly when I climbed down steep inclines or stairs, when I lifted loads that weren't especially heavy and, of course, when I picked up and carried my little grandchildren. My youngest grandchild is three and whenever I pick her up I have to go change my absorbent pad. It also happened during the dancing that I loved so much. I avoid dancing now because I know just how unpleasant it is afterwards. But for me, the worst season is winter. Even a mild bout of the flu, with coughing and sneezing, makes me feel as if I'm constantly "swimming in pee."

This was something that I had hardly ever told anyone apart from my husband, who is my closest friend. I treated it like something people don't talk about—it happens, you change your pad, wash, and move on. When you see something funny on TV, you laugh, you enjoy it, and you go and change your pants. When it happens at home, it's not such a big deal. But if you go out to a show, a comedy, it's unpleasant and ruins your mood, and I find myself impatient to get home.

I've tried all kinds of absorbent pads. By now I'm an expert on the subject. But recently it's gotten so severe that even the best absorbent pads cause chafing, pain, and discomfort. However, I've learned by now how to treat myself with soothing ointments or sitz baths.

When I told my doctor about my urinary incontinence around three years ago, he performed an examination, confirmed what I had told him, and immediately proposed surgery. When I asked about the operation itself, the doctor said that it's a very simple and easy operation in which the lower half of the body is anesthetized with an epidural anesthesia. This is done because the patient must be alert and must cooperate during the operation. But the moment I heard the words epidural anesthesia, I was against the idea. I don't know why. Maybe it's because I'm an older woman, and mainly because I was a nurse for many years, and we longtime nurses are afraid of epidurals. We're members of the "natural childbirth" generation. So I turned down his suggestion and went home to think about it.

About a year later I went back to the doctor for my routine exam and, after hearing that nothing had changed, he again proposed surgery. He claimed that the operation would improve my quality of life and sent me for urodynamic testing to see whether I was a candidate for such an operation. The testing confirmed beyond a doubt that I was a very suitable candidate for such surgery. Once again, I refused. I was also offered all kinds of physiotherapy, but I didn't try it because I thought it was too late for someone in my condition. Physiotherapy is good, but I hadn't heard about any major successes.

A few months ago I saw my doctor again. He was surprised that I wasn't going to have the operation and resume a comfortable, quality life. He added that he was aware of my reservations and said that the operation can now be performed under general anesthesia as well. Although I am aware of the dangers of general anesthesia, it's still extremely tempting. The proposed surgery is performed vaginally. It involves a small incision and supporting the urethra with tape so that it won't disrupt the normal urine flow. The doctor explained to me that the procedure is easy, and that patients can resume their normal activities just two or three weeks after the operation—if the surgery is successful and there are no complications, of course. At the moment, I'm still debating with myself.

By now I have told close family members and my girlfriends, and have found out that some of them have the same problem but behave like me, accepting the situation and getting on with their lives as if urinary incontinence is a decree from on high. I believe that as time passes and medicine and medical research continue to develop, more methods and easy solutions will be found to meet the needs of a large population of women who have come to terms with this unpleasant condition that impairs their quality of life.

CHAPTER 11

Thriving Among the Thistles

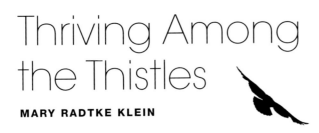

MARY RADTKE KLEIN

EDITOR'S NOTE: Learning to live with or manage incontinence is a good start, but you should know that more may also be possible. Though your life includes a very thorny problem, you needn't just live, you have the potential to thrive. This chapter is about getting unstuck, about carefully picking apart the tangle of concrete problems that hold you back and applying some practical techniques that can help you find workable solutions. Some simple tactics are described to help you boost the creativity you use in problem solving. Add to that ideas for thoughtful planning around some of the most common problems and, with practice, your incontinence can usually begin to slip into the background of a busy life.

How often have you heard someone say "if you do what you've always done, you'll get what you always got"? With incontinence, people find that they may become depressed, fearful, embarrassed, isolated, angry—you know the list. Just listen to the life experiences recounted by the individuals who have contributed to this book. But each one of them found a new path for himself or herself. They each came to a point where they defied the negative emotions and tried something different that moved the quality of their life forward.

It is easy to feel discouraged and frustrated when dealing with incontinence, but it is also truly possible to thrive. Knowing where to find just the right protective garment may not boost your caché at the next neighborhood association meeting, but the same skills that help you live successfully with incontinence can enhance almost every other aspect of your life. Strategic thinking, creativity, no-nonsense planning, resourcefulness, and good communication skills are assets at home, at work, or in any social setting. Another chapter in this book talks about developing resilience, the characteristic that helps us, despite formidable adversity, move forward or get back up after we've taken a blow. You might think about some of the following strategies, tips, and techniques as building blocks to help develop or improve your resilience. The objective is to develop skills to change the way you operate in the world. The goal is to move urinary or fecal incontinence from the focal issue in your life to the status of a problem that you manage confidently like you do so many others.

For many individuals, incontinence is still a painful obstacle rather than a simple challenge. It can be an overwhelming, interconnected nest of dilemmas. One issue often seems to be compounded by another. The magnitude of the barriers and their pervasive influence on daily life sometimes makes the frustrations seem insurmountable. This chapter will encourage you to break this problem apart and name some individual challenges. It will offer some tips, but more importantly, it will suggest some skills that can move you from painful frustration to confronting a specific challenge with a plan of attack.

Strategies

Incontinence of the bowel or bladder has a wide variety of causes and is experienced in many different ways by different people. Some people may have frequent and often unpredictable problems and challenges; others may have trouble less often or with clear regularity. Individual issues can vary from feeling minor to annoying to catastrophic. The information below certainly won't address every single problem, but here are some ideas to get you started.

Labeling the Problem and Breaking it Apart

Whether you are striving to solve an individual problem or simply hope to improve your creativity, a fundamental step is to isolate, name, and describe the target problem as specifically as possible. Important problems are usually emotionally loaded. Anxiety, anger, depression, and emotional fatigue can keep our attention focused on the tangled nature of a problem and prevent us from identifying individual pieces that we might be able to fix. Confidence is often built through a series of small victories. Begin your problem solving by stepping back from the emotion and creating a concrete definition of the problem itself.

Some problem solving experts suggest picking the easiest problem to work on first; others opt for a couple of related but modest problems as a starting point. Still others recommend tackling the biggest, most fearful or annoying problem, putting all of your energy into it and getting it out of the way. Any of these options is fine, but whichever you choose, try to clearly isolate, name, and define the problem in objective, behavioral terms.

Defining the Problem

Writing forces you to define the reality and helps narrow the scope of the problem. Get a pen and some paper and try writing down what you see as the problem, specific to incontinence.

Here's an example:
"I can never go out without having a problem with leakage."

Look at the problem statement above and ask if <u>all</u> of its elements are true—they are probably not. Read and examine the statement word by word. Do you have trouble every time you go out? Step one, eliminate the all-encompassing words like *every, always, all, constantly, never, none.* Try to remember the specifics of the last few times you had trouble when you went out. Make a list. Are there any patterns, common threads related to time, persons, places, or things? Let's say "Karen's" name keeps coming up; rewrite the problem with this more concrete information:
"I've had a problem with moderate leakage the last three times I went to dinner at Karen's house."

Can you see how the two problem statements above are different? Maybe the times you had trouble involved a range of circumstances. See if there are any common, recurring elements associated with problem incidents: time, people, places, type of activity, weather. A recurring element may reveal a pattern or an adjustable circumstance and lead you to a significant insight. Defining a problem in concrete terms gives you tangible elements to begin to examine and manipulate.

Now, without a lot of analyzing, make a quick list of problems that are troubling you. Then pick one that you'd like to work on and write it down as a draft problem statement. Examine the statement and rewrite it until it is composed of concrete elements you can work with.

Draft Problem Statement: _____
_____
_____
_____

Concrete Problem Statement: _____
_____
_____
_____

Don't Rush to Fix It, Break It Apart
Every act of creation is first an act of destruction. —Pablo Picasso

Once you've defined the problem, it's tempting to try to apply a fix. If you do that, you may rob yourself of an opportunity to find a more creative or effective solution. Think about the emotions we bring to a frustrating problem. We're fed up, we want to get this solved once and for all, we sometimes feel like we've tried everything, or that the problem is so overwhelming it's unsolvable. These are not emotional states that contribute to open-minded creativity.

It may seem counter-intuitive, but before you rush to a solution, try to break the problem apart. Identifying the elements on paper may help you distance yourself from the emotions and see a new way to approach the problem.

On a piece of paper, you can make space for several boxes or lists. Label them People, Places, Time, Things, Activities, and maybe Miscellaneous. Let's use the following problem statement: *I am getting up every night to urinate (or I am awakened by a loss of urine), then I have trouble falling back to sleep and I'm tired the next day.*

What are the elements in this problem?

People	Places	Time
Myself Dog Kids	Bedroom Bed Bathroom Also happens when I travel	Happens almost every night Bed at 11 PM Wake around 3 AM Get up 6:30 AM
Things	**Activities**	**Miscellaneous**
Bed Bed covers/ pillows Nightgown Absorbent product Liquids, none after 10 PM Medication before bed Clock Radio	Dress for bed Brush teeth Take medication Use an intermittent catheter Read sometimes Fall asleep to radio Go into bathroom to urinate or change Can't fall back to sleep	Like it cool in room

You can see how these lists might grow and reveal elements that trigger ideas. A variety of approaches might suggest themselves.

This example mimics a real-life situation. Doing this exercise called attention to the medications being taken right before bedtime. Because some medications can stimulate urination or urine production, the person involved chose to investigate that path. He questioned the doctor, who changed the time the medication was taken, and in this case, the problem improved significantly.

Notice, the word "solution" wasn't used above. The problems you face are not like arithmetic. There is rarely one right answer. Expect that not every well-thought-out strategy will solve a problem. You may have to pick yourself up and try a different path. But you've developed a technique for distancing yourself from paralyzing, negative emotions, you've learned something from a failed try, and you have given yourself relevant pieces of information to work with. You're on your way to being resilient and successful.

Try this technique with the problem statement of your own.

Working Problem Statement: _____

_____

_____

_____

People	Places	Time
Things	Activities	Miscellaneous

Cornerstone of Creativity

Creativity hardly sounds like a topic to be found in a book on incontinence, but creativity is a tool that supports resilience. Creativity helps you make the leap from just surviving to thriving. Begin by understanding that, in terms of resilience, some people are naturally gifted, but the rest of us can develop the skill.

Each of us usually starts with ideas formed from our own experience. That's a fairly limited pool. Unless we're naturally creative, we often carry around and usually apply preconceived and unhelpful patterns of thinking:

■ That's not practical
■ That's not logical
■ I could never do that
■ He/she/people would think I…
■ It would cost too much
■ That's weird
■ Herman would never agree
■ That won't work…

Creativity's first demand is that we suspend judgment. Judgment comes later. The initial focus is on generating ideas. Use stored and forgotten experiences and information, use unassociated elements to provoke new ideas, and draw upon the ideas of others whenever possible (use good friends, professionals, the Internet).

The best way to have a good idea is to have lots of ideas. —Linus Pauling, Nobel Laureate

Brainstorming is a common technique for generating ideas. To be effective, the goal is to generate as many ideas as possible. In this case, the ideal is quantity not quality:

■ Generate as many ideas as possible.
■ Involve others if possible.
■ Do not judge or evaluate ideas. Write every one down. Don't think about an idea being either good or bad.
■ Humor helps.

If we go back to the problem of waking at night, we can look at all of its elements (people, places, time, things) and just start manufacturing ideas about things we might change. Now look at the list and start picking out ideas that sound plausible. In addition to generating ideas, this kind of a process prevents you from investing all your energy and faith in finding "the solution." It helps to remind you that there's probably no single, right, complete solution.

Try it with your problem statement.

Brainstorming Solutions

Leave a night light on

Keep the room warmer

Wear looser night clothes

Don't drink liquids after 6 PM

Kick the dog off the bed

Make time for a brief nap every afternoon

Sleep on the couch / another bed

See if there's a medicine to keep me from urinating at night

Change medications

Wear a heavier/different absorbent product

Read twenty minutes before trying to sleep again

Use an intermittent catheter to empty the bladder after I finish reading

Keep a urinal by the bed

Don't turn on the light in the bathroom when I get up

Put earplugs in when I go back to bed

Brush teeth earlier

Think about being a dog falling asleep on a cozy cushion

Listen to soft music or a boring book on tape through iPod/Walkman earbuds

Set alarm to get up at 2 AM and try to urinate

Get a night-shift job

Other Creativity Tricks

Ask how would "X" solve this problem?

- Nancy Regan
- Margaret Thatcher
- Bill Gates
- The Three Stooges
- James Bond
- Darth Vader (Star Wars)
- My hero
- A miner
- An astronaut
- A mountain climber
- Lady Gaga

Find a general interest magazine, novel, or newspaper and randomly point to five to seven words, or try to Google a "random word list" on the Internet and find a small number of random words. Write them down on a sheet of paper next to you as you are doing your brainstorming. Though the words seem unrelated to your challenge, see if you can use them to spark an idea.

Disrupt your thinking if you are struggling with a problem, don't keep trying harder. Stop and write a poem about love or auto racing. What if you're not a poet? Do something else distracting.

If you are addressing the same problem for the fifth time, spend time congratulating yourself on your perseverance and resilience. Then, consider reframing the problem statement to see if it gives you a fresh outlook.

Use substitution. If you have a great idea but it's too expensive, takes too much time, or might be considered rude or selfish, what elements could you change or substitute to salvage the idea?

Don't let the excellent stand in the way of the good. As you generate ideas, don't discard an idea because it doesn't solve the whole problem. It may be an imperfect solution, but it may provide an increment of quality improvement in your life. Implementing it may lead you to new insights.

Set a deadline. This sounds more like a restriction than a tool to promote creativity. For the procrastinators among us, however, a deadline may provide inspiration. Can you create a sense of urgency (i.e., pressing importance) that will spur you to creative action? Set a dinner date with Karen. Put a down payment on a long weekend trip. Deny yourself your favorite candy until you have a clear problem statement written down. Don't think about doing something, strip your mind of thoughts and emotions and "Just do it!"

In summary, this kind of problem solving requires:
- Naming and defining the problem in a written statement
- Breaking apart the elements in the problem situation
- Applying riotous creativity to generating possible responses
- Assembling a new approach from the pieces you've created

These are techniques for wrestling with individual, specific circumstances that challenge you. You'll want to tackle problems one at a time as you have the need and energy. The good news is that you will find that you become better as you practice these skills. You will be amazed at the skill you develop and the confidence you build from your success.

Planning

Planning is different from individual problem solving. It is an ongoing behavior that integrates what you know with what you want or need to do day to day. For anyone who lives with a chronic health problem, planning is essential to quality of life.

One of the most successful planners out there is a young professional who was born with an anal anomaly that created chronic fecal incontinence. He'll tell you that he learned to thrive by thinking of himself as "an undercover secret agent," always looking ahead, finding ways to blend in, keeping his very significant impairment "undercover." Today he has, in his words "come out of the closet" and is becoming a very public spokesperson for those with incontinence. But for years it was conscious planning and creativity that helped him meet his then-objective of keeping his incontinence well below the radar.

The Practice of Planning

When life is busy and chronic health issues compound its complexity, we often operate on automatic pilot, plowing through from one task to the next. Then we collapse. The gentleman mentioned earlier in this section said, "If you're incontinent, and want to blend into the flow of life you've got to plan, plan, plan." Using his James Bond model, you plan for known dangers and the unexpected with skill and an arsenal of information.

The Franklin Covey enterprise has made a fortune in the United States by teaching people how to be effective through planning. Two of their fundamental strategies are:
■ Begin with the end in mind
■ Commit to planning

If you don't know where you are going, you are unlikely to get there. This is true whether you are just trying to get through the week or are struggling with an individual problem. If you are not clear about what you want and don't take the time to plan for the accomplishment, you are likely to end up disappointed and frustrated. If you are living with incontinence, you have an added hurdle. You need to know yourself, your environment, and related resources in a level of detail that most other people don't have to think about.

As you plan, you'll want to think about the number and type of obligations and activities you have for a given day, week, or event. How do you use your time? What is your energy level, your tolerance for stress? How many people, animals, projects do you have commitments to? Can you describe the rhythm of your day; morning, afternoon, evening, night, weekends? Review the environments you move in, their related safety, social expectations, travel requirements, and expenses. Give these elements enough thought that you can easily build that information into planning a day, a week, a weekend, a trip, an event. You will find yourself incorporating this detail into the specific problem solving you do. How you choose to address a problem may be dependent on these elements. If your energy is best in the early morning, planning to grocery shop after work is less likely to be successful.

Finally, armed with this information, commit the time to planning. Ask "What do I need to do, or to accomplish?" For each activity, ask what or how do I need to prepare? How much time will this take? What are the elements I can manipulate? Finally, when is the best time or what is the best sequence in which to accomplish this?

For some people, going to the grocery store may require special preparation and planning to ensure a successful outing. Those plans might include:

- Timing this for early morning Sunday when energy is high and shoppers are few.
- Laying out a lightweight, quick-dry pair of dark pants that can be easily slipped off, along with other clothes for the morning.
- Having a shopping list arranged section by section for the grocery store to shorten the time spent.
- Knowing where the grocery store's restroom is and if it's available to the public, or if you need permission or a key to use it.
- Asking for help carrying groceries if lifting heavy bags can cause leakage. Many stores are happy to help you load your groceries in your car.
- Packing your "stand-by" handbag, tote, carryall, briefcase, or messenger bag with supplies that might be necessary if you have an unexpected need.
- If the length of the trip, the weight of bags, or stepping out into the cold is likely to trigger leakage, park as conveniently as possible and go into the house without bags first. Then return for bags once you know you are prepared.

You can see that planning takes several forms. As you practice, the thought patterns and rhythms will become natural and you'll find yourself becoming accomplished in the "tradecraft" (espionage jargon for the set of skills that makes spies successful and keeps them alive as they blend into the routines of the world, never allowing anyone to suspect their secrets).

Common Issues and Ideas

When you are planning, you will call on your own experience. But you will also want to develop a library of new information. There are pitfalls, resources, and tactical strategies that others have uncovered. Successful planning means taking the time to build these into your arsenal.

The following is no exhaustive reference, but simply a starting point to spark ideas and begin your own research.

Energy and Fatigue: It's Just a Matter of Time

Living with incontinence takes extra time. To compound the issue, incontinence may only be one in a series of symptoms that accompany a chronic illness or disability.

It almost goes without saying that you need to track urination and bowel movements enough to determine your individual patterns. But beyond that examine your energy level in general, how it ebbs and flows over the course of a day, a task, or an event. Use this information to plan. Don't hesitate to graciously ask that tasks or appointments be scheduled at a time that will accommodate your needs.

Try to schedule tasks or activities in blocks of time that fit your bladder or bowel patterns and your energy limits. Consolidate errands and delegate when you can. If planning an activity of some length, be sure to anticipate the approximate time when you need to be near a bathroom or back at home. Find a way for others to have some idea about your needs so that they can be taken into account.

> " *There is nothing noble in being superior to some other man. The true nobility is in being superior to our previous self.* "
>
> —*Old Hindu Proverb*

Also, plan breaks and downtime to recharge your battery. Find out if you are a power-napper who is refreshed by a ten to twenty minute snooze.

Be honest with yourself about how much time all the little tasks take. If you are overly optimistic about the speed at which your body and mind can move, all your good planning will be wasted.

The Environment as a Resource and a Barrier

The availability of a bathroom is often critical. Where you regularly shop or do business might depend on the accessibility of a clean restroom. Know where the restroom is in establishments you frequent. Those who have smart-phones and access to the Internet can now download free apps like *Have2P* which provides information on the closest restroom, based on your current location.

Consider where you can find public restrooms. Might they be in public libraries, large chain bookstores, large retail stores (in the U.S., "big box" stores), large clothing or department stores, hotel lobbies, service/gas stations, or chain coffee shops? Although many restrooms are free, it's a good idea to always have some change handy. Walking into stores or restaurants and approaching someone in charge with a request to use the employee or customer bathroom will often work if you look nonthreatening and slightly desperate.

In your bathroom at home you'll want to have handy and discreet storage space for protective products and hygiene and skin care supplies. Assure that supplies of products are kept in place so that they are at hand when needed. Consider floor, shower, and tub surfaces. They should be well sealed so that germs and odors don't accumulate and multiply. These surfaces should also be non-slip so that in the case of unexpected leakage the liquid or a startled response doesn't lead to a fall.

Some people might find an advantage in having a small foot stool or box that raises their knees slightly above 90° when seated on the toilet. This can help straighten the anal canal and facilitate a bowel movement. Such a foot support can also relieve simple muscle stress if you are seated and your feet cannot rest comfortably to the floor. There is a growing body of research in motility (movement of material in the gut) that may eventually lead to practical, low-tech help for patients.

If you are older, especially if you know you have fragile skin, try not to stay seated on the toilet for a long time. Skin breakdown can be accelerated and your legs can fall asleep, increasing the potential of a fall when you try to get up from a seated position. Installing side bars on the wall or toilet seat can make it easier to use the toilet independently without fear of falling.

Whether you are old or young, it is important to observe the condition of your skin, or have someone you trust observe the condition of your skin. An unobserved reddening can become a skin ulcer in no time at all. Make sure you ask your doctor or nurse to help you monitor your skin condition.

The Little Black Bag

Whether it's a tote, carryall, camera bag, briefcase or messenger bag, sports bag or backpack, you'll want to have an always-at-the-ready carrier for important supplies. A bag with a hook on it allows you to keep it off the floor if there is a hook in a bathroom stall.

Here are a few suggestions for the contents:
- Baby wipes: any brand in the travel-size packs
- Zinc-oxide or petroleum based cream
- Pair of disposable gloves
- Extra briefs or pads: to save space, enclose them in a zip lock bag, sit on the bag to squeeze the air out, and close to create a compressed package
- Extra pair of briefs or pantyhose
- A large zip lock bag to enclose wet or soiled garments: press on the bag to squeeze the air out and compact the soiled contents
- An all-purpose lightweight pair of black pants or a skirt

Expenses

Expenses increase with the need for supplies, medications, skin care products, and briefs, not to mention extra laundry. It's important to budget and not let expenses get away from you without noticing. Here are a couple of ideas to consider.

Find out if your employer offers a flexible spending account as part of the employee benefit package. In the United States, these accounts allow you to contribute pre-tax dollars on a monthly basis to an account that you can spend during the year for uncovered medical expenses and a variety of health care related items including supplies needed to manage medically diagnosed incontinence. Funds deposited to the account must be used within the year or they are lost.

A number of product manufacturers will offer free samples of products. Check Internet sites, contact a wide variety of manufacturers by e-mail or phone and try to get samples. If nothing else, this may be an effective approach for funding the trial and error that is necessary to find the product that works best for you. Local medical supply companies may also have samples or be able to put you in touch with the manufacturer, saving you from buying a large quantity of a product that turns out to be a dud. In the United States, Internet shopping can save on sales tax and provide anonymity with discreetly packaged home delivery.

Investigate the availability of a Diaper Bank in your area. The concept is relatively new and still rare, but these organizations operate much like local Food Banks. They gather supplies of diapers/briefs from manufacturers and volunteer donors. They arrange for the storage and sorting of the products and then make them available to end users through a variety of community organizations. If you cannot find one locally, contact the Simon Foundation. Or, if you have some experience in community development, you might want to find out more about how such a Bank can be developed in your community.

Products

Remember that protective undergarments come in a wide array of styles, shapes, fits, fabrics, weights, and levels of absorbency. The product really needs to be suited to the individual, the type of incontinence, and the particular requirement the consumer needs to meet (protection during a dressy social event or protection during sleep). It might be best to begin, or resume, your search by talking to a continence nurse or contacting a medical supplier. Follow the suggestion above about seeking samples. There is much more on products in Chapter 10.

Accidents

It is an imperfect world and nothing feels more imperfect than the leakage of urine or feces. But, it will happen. So plan for the best and be prepared for the worst.

As you undertake all of the problem solving and planning mentioned earlier, you might want to think about how the following ideas fit into your strategies.

Dress in clothing that is least likely to show stains. Look for fabrics that can be spot washed and dried quickly.

> *"Having a low opinion of yourself is not 'modesty'. It's self-destruction. Holding your uniqueness in high regard is not 'egotism'. It's a necessary precondition to happiness and success.* **"**
> *—Bobbe Sommer*

Today a man can easily carry a small bag/clutch or messenger bag (nice if it has a loop on the end for hanging) with extra underwear and/or an extra absorbent product or pad compacted and sealed in a zip lock bag. A travel pack of wipes and a zip lock for soiled garments may complete the kit, or you might add some disposable gloves and protective ointment. Women might pack similar appropriate items.

Odor

Odor is often a worry, but the worry often exceeds the real cause for concern, especially if you follow some simple guidelines.

Keep your body clean and fresh. Bathe or shower frequently, including after exercise. Use gentle products that won't irritate your skin and pay particular attention to cleaning between your legs and down your inner thighs. Use a moisture barrier cream to protect your skin from exposure to urine or feces.

Use only protective products that fit snugly. A close fit will keep urine or fecal leakage contained. If you are concerned about the fit of a product you like in other respects, consider a snug mesh over-pant that will conform to your body.

When you experience leakage, attend to it immediately and change the soiled pad, pant, or brief even if the leakage is minor. Then carefully cleanse yourself, including your inner thighs. Use alcohol free wipes and a moisture barrier cream to prevent skin irritation. Creams might contain petroleum jelly, paraffin, lanolin, zinc oxide, or cocoa butter. Your continence nurse or pharmacist will have up-to-date recommendations.

If the soiled product is washable, seal it in a zip lock bag to bring home and wash as soon as possible. If it's disposable, seal it in a zip lock bag for immediate disposal (these should not be flushed, but disposed of in garbage containers). Wet or soiled absorbent products or clothes need to be in a sealed container or a bucket with a lid until washed or disposed of so that odor is contained.

Drinking insufficient liquids can result in concentrated urine and strong odor. Drink plenty of water during the day.

Some foods have the reputation for causing changes in urine odor: strong coffee, onions, garlic, asparagus, and some fatty meats. Foods that produce gas may increase the odor in the stool. One by one, try eliminating these foods from your diet for several days and see if you notice a change in the smell of your urine or stools.

You might ask your doctor about deodorizing tablets. Several are sold under the brand names Derifil, Nullo, Devrom, and Chlorofresh in the United States. Vitamin C has also been reported to help, but some people find that citrus juice irritates the bladder.

Finally, the odor of urine and stool do not always wash out of fabrics easily. Several writers recommend spot washing with one part white vinegar to two parts water; as always, try the mixture on an inconspicuous part of clothing first to assure color fastness. It is also suggested that you add either baking soda or white vinegar to your wash, adding an extra cold water rinse afterward. Check the package for a phone number and you may be able to call the detergent manufacturer to determine a safe proportion. For a persistent odor without an apparent source, the use of a black light is said to make the stain glow. (Google: black light urine.)

Your best detector is a trusted friend. Let that person know about your concern and check in with them periodically just to let them know you are serious about wanting to be alerted if they ever smell a hint of unpleasant odor when they are with you or in your home.

Summary

"Begin with the end in mind." The concepts in this chapter have suggested that you define problems in a concrete way, that you break them down into component parts, and apply a healthy measure of creativity to problem solving. You've been encouraged to plan event by event, by knowing yourself and learning what you can from outside resources.

Make the choice to thrive—you deserve to as much as any person. You may have been confronted with a modest or a profound challenge, but you do have a choice in how you respond to it. Try some of these techniques and strategies. Don't allow yourself to be overwhelmed, but simply choose to make a start. Begin step by step and you will move incontinence from a focal issue in your life to a problem that you manage with confidence. You can learn to be creative and resilient. You can thrive.

Resources

Elder Care often involves care related to incontinence. The challenge of incontinence affects older people and those who care for them in many different ways. The University of Florida has an excellent list of resources, called AlzOnline, targeted to the needs of older people and their helpers. Much of the information applies even if Alzheimer's is not the cause of incontinence. The site has links to information on several products and strategies.
www.alzonline.phhp.ufl.edu/en/reading/tet_incontinence.php

MedicineNet is another large website with credible clinical information. It describes its information as doctor-produced. Enter terms such as "incontinence," "urinary incontinence," or "fecal incontinence" in the search box, or click the "Diseases & Conditions" tab and use the search term box or drill down through topics on the page below.
www.medicinenet.com

My Story

MISSY LAVENDER, USA

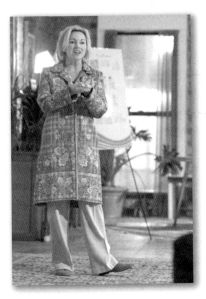

My journey in bladder control and pelvic health began abruptly after the birth of my first child eleven years ago. I was an active, healthy, fit, forty-year-old mother who, in retrospect, experienced the "perfect storm" of childbirth—at least if you intend to become a patient in this arena. My ten-pound son was born with the use of forceps and a very aggressive episiotomy after I pushed for three and a half hours and one of the doctors tried to help by pushing on my stomach to get him to descend. All those factors—my age, forceps, episiotomy, long second-stage labor—led to me becoming an incontinence patient with third-degree prolapse, pelvic pain, and sexual dysfunction.

To say that I was unprepared for this outcome after a model pregnancy was an understatement. When I stood up the morning after my son's birth and something was running out of me that I couldn't identify (I knew it wasn't blood), I rang the nurse frantically. I thought it was amniotic fluid (that's how unprepared I was!). She cleaned me up, patted me on the back, and said, "This is perfectly normal after a forceps delivery." What? "That you would lose control of your bladder," she added. Well, maybe to her it was "normal," but I didn't recall my obstetrician ever mentioning lack of bladder control as a possible outcome of a vaginal delivery.

I left the hospital wearing a super-thick pad, which I continued to wear for six weeks as nothing improved. Both my infant son and I were in the equivalent of diapers. At my six-week appointment I was an emotional wreck and broke down in tears in my doctor's office. She left and went out to check with her partner; when she came back, she patted me on the back (again!) and assured me that everything would be fine. "Go home, give it six months, and do your Kegels," was her advice.

So that's what I tried to do, and in four months, when absolutely nothing had improved and I was still wearing those thick pads, my depression over this new condition and my wildly out of control body led me to make a very fortunate phone call to my good friend who is a psychiatrist. I begged her to put me on an antidepressant. Fortunately, she took the time to try to understand *why* I wanted medication.

"I know you think you need this medicine," she said, "but what you really need is to go see this doctor; she is a urogynecologist," and she gave me her name and number. Here is where I got lucky. Research shows that women cope with symptoms of bladder control for an average of seven years before they bring it up to their doctor and it takes an average four times of them doing so before they receive "treatment"—whatever that turns out to be. I clearly was more aggravated and concerned than the "average" patient and I luckily asked the *right* health care provider who got me quickly and efficiently to the *right* physician.

During my first visit to the urogynecologist she stunned me by sharing the fact that half of her patients were similar to me—older, first time moms who had had episiotomies, forceps, and long second-stage labor—and then she added this comment when I told her about my obstetrician's advice to "go home and do my Kegels." "Telling you to go home and do your Kegels is like telling an athlete who has torn a muscle to go to the gym and work it out—it's not going to happen. You have about 25% of your pelvic floor that will not do anything."

When I recovered from that shocking fact, we got down to discussing my recovery protocol, which included a combination of devices (a pessary and an electrical stimulation unit), biofeedback and physical therapy, plus appropriate exercise and nutrition. I learned a great deal in the two years between baby number one and baby number two. I learned by talking to my friends and my mom's friends, and women in the Starbuck's line, and found there is so much that we don't know about our pelvises and our pelvic health. I kept hearing, "Well, yeah, I have that... but isn't that part of... having a baby/being a woman/getting older... or doesn't it just go away?" It was during this period that the idea took root for doing something to close the gap between what I knew was possible and available for women like me, and the knowledge base of the general population of women.

I ultimately had full pelvic reconstructive surgery and was further energized to "do something" by my wonderfully capable surgeon's post-op recommendation for exercise, which was to "resume my normal activities"—period. No coaching, no physical therapy prescription, no "do's and don'ts," just a simple "resume normal activities." Being an active woman in my late forties, with a hip-to-hip abdominal scar and the fervent wish to never leak again, I could not settle for that blanket statement. I put together a team comprised of a physical therapist, a pelvic floor physical therapist, and a tremendous prenatal/postpartum fitness expert and proceeded to rehab wonderfully from my surgery; eventually getting back to running twice a week (while still wearing my pessary, just in case).

At this point I knew that women in America (and everywhere) needed more—more information, more coaching, more wellness, and more permission to understand this part of their bodies. They needed to learn about their pelvises, what's inside there, how things work, what life-stages are important for pelvic health, what can go wrong, and what they can do to mitigate or prevent things from really going wrong. Maybe most importantly, they needed to know who in the health care system would listen, understand, and effectively treat them if they did experience issues around pelvic health.

I founded the Women's Health Foundation in 2004 with a simple mission, "To improve the pelvic health and wellness of women and girls." We believe strongly that sometimes it's about "changing the world, one pelvic floor at a time." The Women's Health Foundation is committed to giving women the knowledge and the power they need to seek appropriate health care and to help drive policy and research in this important area.

As for my own pelvic health, I always say I'm better and that is good! I can run, with my handy support device (my pessary), I do my pelvic floor exercises, I make decisions about what I eat and drink to lessen that "gotta go" feeling, and I talk—a lot—to other women about their bodies. I love what I do and I know we are changing the world!

A Word About Prevention

You are probably wondering why a section on prevention would be included in a book for people who are already faced with the challenges of incontinence. For most people, prevention means taking steps to see that something never happens in the first place (termed "primary prevention"). However, prevention can be more elaborately defined to include, for instance, preventing incontinence from worsening or causing complications (such as skin problems). Steps which are taken after a health issue has already arisen are referred to as secondary prevention.

For many people, finding ways to manage incontinence and taking steps that will help to prevent worsening, or to regain some control over the bladder or bowel, provides a renewed sense of power and well-being. This is important, because after coming to terms with the fact that you have incontinence (and it's not going away), you may feel that you have lost control over your body. Taking positive action to prevent further problems can change that perception.

Earlier chapters in this book about bowel and bladder function also include, in much more detail, the ideas for reducing the risk of your incontinence worsening, which are summarized here. The concept of prevention cannot be stressed enough. Until medical science is able to cure all incontinence, there are many things that can be done to lessen incontinence. Giving your attention to secondary prevention now, will in turn also lesson incontinence's impact on the quality of your life in the future.

At the Simon Foundation for Continence's International Conference for the Prevention of Incontinence (1997), 42 internationally recognized experts in the field from eleven countries came together in England to explore what was currently known about the prevention of urinary incontinence; to develop recommendations for Healthy Bladder Habits; and to formulate recommendations for avenues of further research about prevention. Although these experts clearly recognized that there were things that could be done for both primary and secondary prevention of incontinence, it was not until more recently that health professionals have started to help their patients to focus on prevention.

Preventing a deterioration of your incontinence is a multi-faceted task. Because prevention is not only important, but also possible, this postscript will provide you with a review of the numerous ways available for improving incontinence or preventing it from becoming worse.

The Importance of Strengthening the Pelvic Floor Muscles

One of the keys to continence involves strengthening the pelvic floor muscles which support the organs and muscles involved in maintaining bladder and bowel control. The pelvic floor is not a rigid platform, but a strong, flexible muscular structure, often described as a hammock. Normal bladder function in both men and women is difficult to maintain without the strength and support of your pelvic floor muscles.

The chapter on urinary incontinence explains the purpose of pelvic floor exercises (often referred to as Kegel exercises after Dr. Kegel who first described them in the 1940s), and offers a clear explanation as to how to do them. This may be all you need to get started. However, if you are like most people you may be unsure if you are doing the exercises correctly or you may even believe that you are, when you are not. This last situation is most unfortunate, because when you see no improvement (due to the fact that you are not doing the exercises correctly) you will in all likelihood abandon your efforts. Happily, when done correctly these exercises might be a great help to you.

The good news is that all of this frustration can be avoided by checking if you are doing the exercises correctly by trying to stop your urine flow mid-stream. If you can stop or slow the flow, you are using the right muscle. Concentrate on what that feels like—it is a pelvic floor contraction. However, do not do this regularly as you can end up not emptying the bladder properly. Another way to check is by trying to squeeze and feeling if anything moves. Both sexes should feel a pucker-up around the anus (back passage). Women can also feel a squeeze inside the vagina and men should notice a pulling up behind the scrotum.

You can also ask your physician, nurse, or physical therapist to physically check to see that you are contracting and relaxing the correct muscles. Your health professional will not only help you locate the correct muscles to exercise, but they, or one of their colleagues, can also use other methods (such as biofeedback) to teach you to do these exercises correctly. Another alternative is electrical stimulation (E-stim), which exercises your muscles for you. E-stim causes your muscles to contract and relax using a very low electrical current. With determination, nearly everyone can find a way to strengthen their pelvic floor muscles, a good first step in preventing a worsening of your incontinence. In addition, doing the exercises correctly is also taking a step that offers the hope of improvement. See page 61 for more details on doing the exercises.

Secondary Prevention of Urinary Incontinence

Today there is more attention to, and research about, prevention. Some suggestions have scientific findings to substantiate the theory that they help to improve or prevent the worsening of incontinence. Other suggestions are what health professionals call "anecdotal," meaning that many individuals have reported that the suggestion has been of help to them. In addition to "proven" methods of prevention, anecdotal ideas (which may or may not draw the attention of scientific researchers in the future) may also be worth trying in order to determine if they help you.

Stopping smoking can help because nicotine can irritate the bladder. Also, chronic coughing caused by smoking may cause stress urinary incontinence.

Maintaining a healthy weight will put less pressure on your bladder. Even a 5% to 10% weight loss has been shown to make a difference.

Determine the proper amount of fluid intake that is right for your body. Find a balance, not too much or too little, by drinking when you are thirsty and checking to see that your urine is not too dark, but rather a pale yellow.

Avoid bladder irritants in your diet, first by learning what is known about the foods and drinks that irritate the bladder (such as caffeine, alcohol, highly spiced food, etc.) and then, one by one, eliminating them from your diet. If you see no improvement, then simply resume eating or drinking that particular item and move on to test the next one on your list. Also check the labels on over-the-counter medications you are taking to be sure they do not contain caffeine.

Keep your bowels regular and avoid constipation. Straining to have a bowel movement can weaken the pelvic muscles.

Try substituting low-impact exercises—activities in which one foot is always on the floor—rather than participating in high-impact activities such as running and high-impact aerobics because these exercises may further weaken the pelvic floor ligaments if they are already weak as they cannot withstand these forces for prolonged periods.

Never ignore symptoms of BPH (benign prostatic hypertrophy) such as urgency, frequency, difficulty starting the urine stream, or a weak urine stream. These changes in urination may be a result of an enlarged prostate gland in men that is pressing upon and narrowing the urethra and causing the bladder to have to work harder to expel the urine. Eventually the bladder muscle simply "gives up" and overflow incontinence results. Overflow incontinence is when urine dribbles from the bladder without your feeling the sensation of bladder fullness. Intervening in time with prostate enlargement can prevent this type of incontinence.

Secondary Prevention of Fecal Incontinence

Working to re-establish bowel control also means working to strengthen the pelvic floor muscles, as they support this area of your body too. In addition, understanding how the bowel moves the digested food through your system will help you to train your bowels. Following are some prevention tips:

Do not skip breakfast because the bowel is stimulated when you wake up in the morning and further by eating and drinking. You can take advantage of this natural awakening of the bowel each day and try to <u>empty the bowel about twenty to thirty</u> minutes after breakfast. Try to make sure your <u>bowel is empty</u> before you start the rest of your day.

> " *The biggest troublemaker you'll probably ever have to deal with, watches you from the mirror every morning.* "
>
> —*Anonymous*

Learn to use the muscles in your abdomen to move your bowels rather than straining, which risks weakening your pelvic floor muscles.

Experiment with fiber in your diet to understand if you have better control with a diet low in fiber or with a diet high in fiber.

Stop smoking because nicotine stimulates the bowel as well as the bladder

Finding an over-the-counter aid that works for you among suppositories, enemas, laxatives, and anti-diarrhea medications might take time and experimentation. However, it may be time well spent if you can find an aid that allows you to choose when your bowel will empty.

Watch your weight because there is some scientific evidence that heavier people are more prone to bowel incontinence.

You Are Never Too Old, and It Is Never Too Late

Did you know that Winston Churchill was 65 when he became Prime Minister of Britain; Claude Monet was 74 when he started painting his celebrated panel of water lilies; Jessica Tandy won her first Oscar at age eighty (for "Driving Miss Daisy"); and at age 89 Frank Lloyd Wright completed his work on the Guggenheim Museum? Like these examples of accomplishments in the late decades of life, you have the ability at every age to work with your body to obtain maximum function.

It is true that aging, especially in the upper years, can make physical challenges more difficult to tackle, yet preventing or slowing possible deterioration is far from impossible. It is important to recognize that some bladder changes are age-related. For instance, bladder sensation may change with age, and bladder capacity is often diminished. In working on secondary prevention these changes may have to be taken into account for your strategy to be successful.

Another challenge for many older adults is night time voiding. A good night's sleep can become harder to obtain as we age and often the two issues (sleep and incontinence) are interconnected. A bladder that behaves properly at night can mean increased sleep. Following are a few of the things you can do to prevent sleep disruption:

A nap during the day of one or two hours, with your feet elevated, helps to increase urine output during daytime hours, leaving less fluid build-up in the body to be excreted at night. You can also reduce swelling and fluid retention in your legs by wearing support stockings during the day.

Make the bathroom the last stop before going to bed so that you start the night with an empty bladder.

Ask your doctor about the timing of taking medications such as diuretics ("water tablets"). It might be a simple matter to switch to taking this medication in the morning instead of the evening.

Understand the effect of medications on your bladder and be aware that blood pressure drugs, cold remedies, diuretics, antidepressants, pain medications, and sleeping pills may all have an effect. Be sure to discuss all your options and alternatives with your pharmacist and/or doctor.

Reduce fluid intake after 6 p.m., and if you have medications that should be taken at bedtime, unless you are instructed to take them with lots of fluids, take these pills with a small amount of water.

Diagnostic Re-checks and Second Opinions

Annual physicals or check-ups are routine for many people, and your incontinence should be re-evaluated on a routine basis too. This is because your incontinence may change over time, and therefore the possibility of the occurrence of underlying health issues should be carefully monitored. Also, your management strategies may need to be modified to meet changing circumstances.

A second opinion regarding your incontinence is also a good idea. It never hurts to feel more educated about our bodies and health, and to see if there might be something new and different offered by another specialist. Having access to specialty nurses is also extremely helpful. Some countries, like the UK, Canada, and Japan, have Nurse Continence Advisors. Depending on the country, these nurses may work in the community. Nurse practitioners, geriatric nurse practitioners, wound, ostomy, continence nurses, and urology nurses all have special knowledge regarding incontinence which might be of help to you.

Knowledge Powers Prevention

Keeping abreast of new information on incontinence goes hand in hand with prevention. Keeping up with new findings, including new products and devices that come into the marketplace, is easier now than ever. Hopefully, you have access to a computer that has Internet at home or at a local public library. There are many organizations that provide news, abstracts, and alerts regarding incontinence research findings (see Worldwide Resources). Because today healthcare professionals have to stay abreast of advances in so many areas, it is possible that your doctor or nurse could overlook something that might benefit you. Taking the time now to be the eyes and ears on something that is of the utmost importance to you can only be of benefit to you in the long run.

Hope for the Future

You might be surprised to learn that both the medical profession and industry have not focused on incontinence until relatively recently. For instance, the International Continence Society is celebrating its 40th anniversary as this book goes to press and all of the editors of this book can remember a time not too long ago when absorbent products were not to be found on retail shelves, and medications to treat incontinence did not exist. The fact that so much has changed in a little more than three decades creates hope for what the future can bring to solve this challenge. Doing all you can now to understand and use techniques for prevention at every level will assure you are in the best position to take advantage of the innovations that are sure to come in the future.

In this book we have provided you with resources (pages 199-209), a bibliography (pages 197-198), and a suggested reading list (pages 215-219) so that you will continue to find new management tools that will assist you in the years ahead. In order to keep you constantly informed, the publisher of this book, The Simon Foundation for Continence, has also launched a tandem website for the book (see Worldwide Resources). But perhaps the single most important aspect of prevention, and one that is completely in your hands, is to be your own advocate, constantly seeking the newest information on managing incontinence so that you can have ongoing informed patient – health care practitioner interactions. Be actively involved with the management of your incontinence and never be too shy to discuss new ideas, treatments, and innovations you've learned about with your doctor or nurse.

Bibliography

Chapter 1

Green, Gill. *The End of Stigma? Changes in the Social Experience of Long-Term Illness.* London: Routledge, 2009.

Myers, Kimberly R. "Coming Out: Considering the Closet of Illness." *Journal of Medical Humanities* 2.4 (2004): 255-270.

Tangney, June Price, and Ronda L. Dearing. *Shame and Guilt.* New York: Guilford Press, 2002.

Tracy, Jessica L., Richard W. Robins, and June Price Tangney, eds. *The Self-Conscious Emotions: Theory and Research.* New York: Guilford Press, 2007.

Chapter 2

Garcia, Julie A., Jennifer Crocker, and Jean F. Wyman. "Breaking the Cycle of Stigmatization: Managing the Stigma of Incontinence in Social Interactions." *Journal of Wound, Ostomy & Continence Nursing* 32.1 (2005): 38-52.

Goffman, Erving. *Stigma: Notes on the Management of Spoiled Identity.* Englewood Cliffs: Prentice-Hall, 1963.

Heatherton, Todd F., ed. *The Social Psychology of Stigma.* New York: Guilford Press, 2000.

Olkin, Rhoda. *What Psychotherapists Should Know About Disability.* New York: Guilford Press, 1999.

Chapter 5

Alberti, Robert, and Michael Emmons. *Your Perfect Right: Assertiveness and Equality in Your Life and Relationships.* 8th ed. San Luis Obisco: Impact Press, 2001.

Cash, Thomas F. *The Body Image Workbook: An Eight-Step Program for Learning to Like Your Looks.* 2d ed. Oakland: New Harbinger Press, 2008.

Chapter 8

Berger, Susan A. *Five Ways We Grieve: Finding Your Personal Path to Healing after the Loss of a Loved One.* Boston: Trumpeter, 2009.

Butler, Timothy. *Getting Unstuck: How Dead Ends Become New Paths.* Boston: Harvard Business School Press, 2007.

Edwards, Elizabeth. *Resilience: Reflections on the Burdens and Gifts of Facing Life's Adversities.* New York: Broadway Books, 2010.

Bibliography, *continued*

Frankl, Viktor E. *Man's Search for Meaning.* Trans. Ilse Lasch. Boston: Beacon Press, 2006.

Groopman, Jerome. *Anatomy of Hope: How People Prevail in the Face of Illness.* New York: Random House, 2003.

Reivich, Karen, and Andrew Shatte. *The Resilience Factor: 7 Keys to Finding Your Inner Strength and Overcoming Life's Hurdles.* New York: Broadway Books, 2002.

Worldwide Resources

EDITOR'S NOTE: Keep in mind as you search for information on Internet sites that not all sites are equal: sites are sponsored by product manufacturers, medical centers, consumer groups, or simply interested individuals. Opinions and information may be more or less credible depending upon the source. Ask a friend, check with your health care provider, and compare information from one site to another. Look for a tab or link that's called "About" or "About Us" to learn more about the sponsoring party. Credible sites allow you to see who they are, how they're sponsored, and what their credentials are. Some sites will be directly sponsored by a well-known university or hospital center. Others are private for-profit organizations that may have excellent content and make their money through advertisers who buy well-defined advertising space on their pages.

AUSTRALIA

Continence Foundation of Australia
Level 1
30-32 Sydney Road
Brunswick VIC 3056
Tel: (61) 03 9347 2522
Website: www.continence.org.au
Email: info@continence.org.au

AUSTRIA

Medizinische Gesellschaft fur Inkontinenhilfe Osterreich
Speckbacherstrasse 1 A-6020, Innsbruck
Tel: (43) 512 58 38 03
Fax: (43) 512 58 94 86
Website: www.inkontinenz.at
Email: kontinenz@telering.at

BELGIUM

U-Control vzw (Belgian Association for Incontinence)
Leopoldstraat 24
B-30000 Leuven
Tel: (32) 8161 6455 / (32) 3821 3047

continued on next page

Urobel vzw
De Pintelaan 185
BE-9000 Ghent
Tel: (32) 09 240 27 65
Fax: (32) 09 240 38 89
Website: www.urobel.be

BRAZIL

Brazilian Foundation for Continence Promotion
Email: seabrarios@uol.com.br

CANADA

Canadian Continence Association
P.O. Box 417
Peterborough, Ontario
K9J 6Z3
Tel: (1) 705 750 4600
Fax: (1) 705 750 1770
Website: www.canadiancontinence.ca
Email: help@canadiancontinence.ca

THE CZECH REPUBLIC

Inco Forum
Česká společnost podpory zdraví
Fakultní Thomayerova nemocnice s poliklinikou
Vídeňská 800
140 59 Praha 4
Tel: (420) 261 083 186
Website: www.inco-forum.cz/
Email: kucerova@cspz.cz

DENMARK

Kontinensforeningen (The Danish Association of Incontinent People)
Vester Farimagsgade 6, 1. sal - kontor 1029
1606 Copenhagen V
Tel: (45) 3332 5274
Website: www.kontinens.dk/
Email: info@kontinens.dk

FINLAND

Finnish Continence Club
Contact: pentti.kiilholma@tyks.fi for details

FRANCE

Association d'Aide aux Personnes Incontinentes
5, Avenue du Marechal Juin
92100 BOULOGNE

Tel: (33) 01 46 99 18 99
Fax: (33) 01 46 99 18 85
Email: aapi@9online.fr

GERMANY

Deutsche Kontinenz Gesellschaft e.V.
Friedrich-Ebert-Strasse 124
34119 Kassel
Tel: (49) 561 78 06 04
Website: www.gih.de

Selbsthilfeverband Inkontinenz e.V.
Website: www.selbsthilfeverband-inkontinenz.org/svi_suite/index.php

HONG KONG

Hong Kong Continence Society
c/o Dept of Medicine and Geriatrics United Christian Hospital
130 Hip Wo Street, Kwun Tong
Kowloon
Tel: (852) 2598 4988
Fax: (852) 2598 6720
Website: www.hkcs.hk
Email: postmaster@hkcs.hk

HUNGARY

Inko Forum
Levelezeski cim, Budapest
Pf 701/153, 1399
Tel: (36) 06 80 730 007
Website: www.inkoforum.hu

INDIA

Indian Continence Foundation
c/o Bangalore Kidney Foundation
CA6, 11th Cross, 15th Main
Padmanabhanagar
Bangalore 560010
Website: www.indiancontinencefoundation.org/
Email: icfindia@vsnl.net

INDONESIA

Indonesian Continence Society
Sub Dept of Urogynecology, Dept of OBGYN Medical Faculty of University
Dr. Cipto Margunkusuma Hospital
Tel: (62) 21 392874 392 3632
Fax: (62) 21 392874 3145592
Email: urogyn@centrin.net.id

continued on next page

ISRAEL

National Center for Continence
Rambam Medical Centre
POB-9602
Haifa 31096
Tel: (972) 485 43197
Fax: (972) 484 42098
Email: ig054@hotmail.com

ITALY

Associazione Italiana Donne Medico (AIDM)
Tel: (39) 335 282045/39 065 811390
Website: www.donnemedico.org

The Federazione Italiana INCOntinenti (FINCO)
Segreteria/Presidenza
V.le O Flacco, 24-70124 Bari
Tel: (39) 080 5093389
Fax: (39) 080 5619181
Website: www.finco.org

Fondazione Italiana Continenza (The Italian Continence Foundation)
Via dei Contarini, 7, 201 33 Milano
Email: info@continenza-italia.org

JAPAN

Japan Continence Action Society
103 Juri Heim, 1-4-2 Zenpukuji
Suginami-Ku
Tokyo 1670041
Website: www.jcas.or.jp/
Email: nishimura@jcas.or.jp

KOREA

Korean Continence Foundation
388-1 Dep of Urology Asan Center
Ulsan University College of Medicine
(138-736) Pungnap-2dong, Songpa-gu
Seoul 138-736
Tel: (82) 2 3010 3735
Fax: (82) 2 477 8928
Website: www.kocon.or.kr/
Email: mschoo@amc.seoul.kr

MALAYSIA

Continence Foundation (Malaysia)
c/o University Hospital
Lembah, Pantai

Kuala Lumpur 59100
Tel: (60) 3 7956 4422
Fax: (60) 3 758 6063
Email: lohcs@medicine.med.um.edu.my

MEXICO

Asociación de Enfermedades Uroginecológicas
ACI Mexuci AC
Tel: (52) 53 74 3691

THE NETHERLANDS

Pelvic Floor Netherlands
PO Box 23594
1100EB, Amsterdam
Tel: (31) 20 69 70 304
Fax: (31) 20 69 71 191

Pelvic Floor Patients Foundation (SBP)
Stichting Bekkenbodem Patiënten
Stationspleing
3818 LE Amersfoort
Email: info@bekkenbodem.net
Tel: (31) 900 111999
Website: www.bekkenbodem.net/

Vereniging Nederlandse Incontinentie, Verpleegkundigen (V N I V)
Postbus 1206
3434 CA
Nieuwegein
Tel: (31) 30 606 0053
Fax: (31) 30 608 1312

NEW ZEALAND

New Zealand Continence Association
PO Box 270
Drury 2247
Free Phone HELPLINE 0800 650 659 (in country only)
Website: www.continence.org.nz/
Email: zoe@continence.org.nz

NORWAY

NOFUS (Norwegian Society for Patients with Urologic Diseases)
Øyjordsveien 71
5038 Bergen
Tel: (47) 55 95 35 88 - 55 33 09 30
Fax: (47) 55 33 09 31
Website: www.nofus.no
Email: rofonnes@online.no   *continued on next page*

PHILIPPINES

Continence Foundation of the Philippines
Room 201, #319 Katipunan Road
Loyola Heights, Quezon City 1108
Tel: (63) 2 4333602
Email: dtbolong@skynet.net

POLAND

NTM "Incontinence—To Live a Normal Life"
(The Polish Continence Organization)
13 Erazma Ciolka St.
01-445 Warsaw
Website: www.ntm.pl/
Email: ntm@ntm.pl

UroConti
Website: www.uroconti.pl/

SINGAPORE

Society for Continence
45 Jalan Pemimpin
Foo Wah Industrial Building #09-20
Singapore 577197
Tel: (65) 6798 0337
Fax: (65) 6588 1723
Website: www.sfcs.org.sg/medi_page/site_web_sfcs/common_page.asp
Email: rani.sfcs@pacific.net.sg

SLOVAKIA

Slovakia Inco Forum
P.O. Box 78
850 00 Bratislava
Tel: (421) 2 67 26 73 40
Fax: (421) 2 62 24 06 30
Website: www.incoforum.sk
Email: info@inkoforum.sk

SOUTH AFRICA

Continence Association of South Africa (CASA)
Affiliated to Association of Continence Advice
PO Box 6479
Westgate 1734
Tel: (27) 022 475 9700
Helpline: 072 2108769 (in country only)
Fax: (27) 011 475 8282
Email: casa123@absmail.co.za

SPAIN

Asociación Nacional de Ostomizados e Incontinentes (ANOI)
Salvador Giner, 2
46110 Godella, Valencia
Tel: (34) 96 390 17 70

SWEDEN

SINOBA
Website: www.sinoba.se/
Email: info@sinoba.se

Swedish Urotherapists
Nordensioldsgatan 10
S-413 09, Goteborg
Tel: (46) 31 50 26 39
Fax: (46) 31 53 68 32
Email: birgtha.lindehall@vgregion.se

SWITZERLAND

Schweizerische Gesellschaft für Blasenschwäche
Gewerbestrasse 12
CH-8132 Egg
Tel: (41) 1 994 74 30
Fax: (41) 1 994 74 31
Website: www.inkontinex.ch
Email: info@inkontinex.ch

TAIWAN

Taiwan Continence Society
Division of Urology, Taipei Veterans General Hospital
201 Sec, 2, Shih-Pai Road
Taipei, Taiwan 112
Tel: (886) 2 2871 1132
Fax: (886) 2 2871 1162
Website: www.tcs.org.tw
Email: msuuf@ms15.hinet.net

UNITED KINGDOM

Association For Continence (ACA)
102a Astra House
Arklow Road, New Cross
London SE14 6EB
Tel: (44) 020 8692 4680
Fax: (44) 020 8692 6217
Website: www.aca.uk.com
Email: info@aca.com.uk

continued on next page

Bladder and Bowel Foundation
SATRA Innovation Park
Rockingham Road
Kettering, Northants, NN16 9JH
Counselor Helpline: 0870 770 3246 (in country only)
General enquiries: (44) 01536 533255
Website: www.bladderandbowelfoundation.org
Email: info@bladderandbowelfoundation.org

The Cystitis & Overactive Bladder Foundation
King's Court
17 School Road
Birmingham, B28 8JG
Tel: (44) 0 121 7020820
Website: www.cobfoundation.org/
Email: info@cobfoundation.org

ERIC – Education and Resources for Improving Childhood Continence
Education and Resources for Improving Childhood Continence
36 Old School House, Britannia Road
Kingswood, Bristol BS15 8DB
Helpline: 0845 370 8008 (in country only)
Website: www.eric.org.uk/
Email: info@eric.org.uk

PROMOCON
Burrows House
10 Priestley Road
Wardley Industrial Estate
Worsley, M28 2LY
Tel: (44) 0161 607 8200
Fax: (44) 0161 607 8201
Website: www.promocon.co.uk/aboutpromocon.shtml
Email: promocon@disabledliving.co.uk

St. Mark's Hospital
Website: www.stmarkshospital.org.uk/patient-information-leaflets

THE UNITED STATES OF AMERICA

American College of Gastroenterology
Patient Education and Resource Center
6400 Goldsboro Rd.
Ste. 450
Bethesda, MD 20817
Tel: (1) 301 263 9000
Website: www.acg.gi.org/patients/gihealth/fi.asp

American Urological Association Foundation
1000 Corporate Boulevard
Linthicum, MD 21090
Tel: (1) 410 689 3990
Fax: (1) 410 689 3998
Website: www.urologyhealth.org
Email: auafoundation@auafoundation.org

Continence Central
Website: www.continencecentral.org

Health Central Incontinence Network
Website: www.incontinencenetwork.com

Interstitial Cystitis Association of America (ICA)
100 Park Avenue, Suite 108-A
Rockville, MD 20850
Website: www.ichelp.org
Email: icamail@ichelp.org

National Association for Continence (NAFC)
P.O. Box 1019
Charleston, SC 29402-1019
Tel: (1) 843 377 0900
Fax: (1) 843 377 0905
Website: www.nafc.org/
Email: memberservices@nafc.org

National Institute on Aging (NIA)
Building 31, Room 5C27
31 Center Drive, MSC 2292
Bethesda, MD 20892
Tel: (1) 800 222 2225 (in country only)
TTY: (1) 800 222 4225 (in country only)
Fax: (1) 301 496 1072
Website: www.nia.nih.gov

National Institute of Diabetes and Digestive and Kidney Diseases (NIDDK)
Office of Communications & Public Liaison
NIDDK, NIH
Bldg 31, Rm 9A06
31 Center Drive, MSC 2560
Bethesda, MD 20892-2560
Tel: (1) 301 496 3583
Website: www.niddk.nih.gov

continued on next page

Pull-Through Network
2312 Savoy Street
Hoover, AL 35226-1528
Tel: (1) 205 978 2930
Website: www.PullthruNetwork.org
Email: PTNmail@charter.net

The Simon Foundation for Continence
PO Box 815
Wilmette IL 60091
Tel: (1) 847 864 3913
Fax: (1) 847 864 9758
Website: www.simonfoundation.org/
Email: info@simonfoundation.org

Society of Urologic Nurses and Associates (SUNA)
East Holly Avenue
Box 56
Pitman, NJ 08071-0056
Tel: (1) 888 827 7862 (in country only)
Website: www.suna.org
Email: suna@ajj.com

Us TOO! International Prostate Cancer Survivor Support Groups
5003 Fairview Avenue
Downers Grove, IL 60515
Prostate Cancer Support Helpline: (1) 800 808 7866 (in country only)
Tel: (1) 630 795 1002
Fax: (1) 630 795 1602
Website: www.ustoo.org
Email: ustoo@ustoo.org

Women's Health Foundation
632 W. Deming Place
Chicago, IL 60614-2676
Tel: (1) 773 305 8200
Fax: (1) 773 305 8211
Website: www.womenshealthfoundation.org/

INTERNATIONAL

Innovating for Continence
Website: www.innovatingforcontinence.org

International Continence Society (ICS)
19 Portland Square
Bristol
Bristol BS2 8SJ
England
Tel: (44) 117 9444881
Website: www.icsoffice.org/
Email: info@icsoffice.org

International Foundation for Functional Gastrointestinal Disorders (IFFGD)
PO Box 170864
Milwaukee, WI 53217-8076
USA
Tel: (1) 414 964 1799
Toll-free: (1) 888 964 2001 (in country only)
Website: www.iffgd.org/
Email address: iffgd@iffgd.org

International Painful Bladder Foundation (IPBF)
Burgemeester Le Fèvre de Montignylaan 73
3055 NA Rotterdam
The Netherlands
Tel/fax: (31) 10 4613330
Email: info@painful-bladder.org

Managing Life with Incontinence
Website: www.managinglifewithincontinence.org

World Federation of Incontinent Patients (WFIP)
Website: www.wfip.org/
Email: presidency@wfip.org

Author Biographies

Lesley Dibley, MPhil, RN

Ms. Dibley is a nurse researcher who has worked with Professor Christine Norton (see below) for several years on studies addressing bowel control issues and the ways that these affect peoples' lives. Her interest in peoples' experiences of illness began early on in her nursing career, and she is particularly interested in issues of difference, marginalization, and stigma which affect access to, and uptake of, health care services. She has published several articles and is currently undertaking her PhD exploring the role of stigma in people with inflammatory bowel disease.

Pamela Dubyak, MS

Ms. Dubyak is a doctoral candidate in the Department of Clinical and Health Psychology at the University of Florida where her research focuses on weight management.

Cheryle B. Gartley

Ms. Gartley is Founder and President of The Simon Foundation for Continence. She is the co-author and editor of the first book for the layperson on incontinence, *Managing Incontinence: A Guide to Living with Loss of Bladder Control* (published in English, Spanish, and Japanese). Cheryle has authored articles in journals such as *The Lancet, Urologic Nursing, Exceptional Parent*, and *Social Work Today*. She is the co-founder of the International Continence Society's Continence Promotion Committee and the Canadian Continence Foundation. As a patient advocate Cheryle has lectured throughout the world about incontinence.

Susan Hayward, PCC

Ms. Hayward is a certified Life Coach, graduated from the Falling Awake School of Life Coaching, and holds a Professional Certified Coach (PCC) credential from the International Coach Federation. She is an active member of the non-profit organization One to One Women Coaching Women, where she provides pro bono coaching to clients, and also serves on the Board of Directors. Susan has created several coaching curricula: Life by Design, Coach for Success, and The 10 Critical Conversations to Have with Your Aging Parents. Susan brings to her coaching practice a wealth of experience, having worked with people in a variety of settings over the years. Ms. Hayward was the Program Director of several shelters for homeless families in New York City, taught high school biology, designed a health program for a school for disadvantaged children while living in Colombia, South America, and ran an organic vegetable farm in California for ten years. Susan is fluent in Spanish. She received her BS from the University of Illinois at Urbana-Champaign and her MS from the University of California, Davis. She currently provides individual and group coaching with an emphasis on Elder Care Coaching.

Mary Radtke Klein

Ms. Klein has spent the past thirty years as an advocate, consultant, and trainer interested in affordable health care and quality improvement in long-term care settings. Mary is the author of *The Oregon Nursing Home Guidebook* and served on the Board of Directors of the National Citizens Coalition for Nursing Home Reform, advocating for and shaping significant federal nursing home regulations. She has been actively involved with Oregon's regulators and development companies since the inception of assisted living in Oregon. As a well-respected regional trainer Mary developed programs for administrators, nurses, and other management personnel, focusing on regulatory compliance, person-centered resident services, and creative problem solving. Her programs focus on the design and implementation of resident services based on quality of life values, appropriate assessment, and preference-based service planning.

Diane K. Newman, DNP, ANP-BC, FAAN, BCB-PMD

Dr. Newman is the Co-director of the Penn Center for Continence and Pelvic Health in the Division of Urology at the University of Pennsylvania Medical Center in Philadelphia. She is Adjunct Associate Professor of Urology in Surgery and Research Investigator Senior in the Perelman School of Medicine at the University of Pennsylvania. Her practice involves the evaluation, treatment, and management of urinary incontinence and related problems including the use of catheters and other devices in the management of bladder dysfunction. She is the urology expert consultant to the acute care staff at her university.

Dr. Newman is the Principal Investigator, University of Pennsylvania, *Translating Unique Learning for Incontinence Prevention: The TULIP Project*, R01NR012011, National Institute of Nursing Research, National Institutes of Health. She is co-investigator on the *Pelvic Floor Disorders Network Clinical Sites* (1U10HD069010-01) National Institutes of Health, Eunice Kennedy Shriver National Institute of Child Health and Human Development, The Office of Research on Women's Health study. She was the Chairperson of the 2nd, 3rd, 4th, and 5th Committee on Continence Promotion, Education & Primary Prevention for the International Consultation on Incontinence. She was the Chair of the International Continence Society (ICS) Continence Promotion Committee (2003-2009). She is an internationally known speaker on the topic of urinary incontinence and the use of devices and products for its management. A prolific writer, Dr. Newman has written and presented more than 100 scientific papers, chapters, and articles on the assessment, treatment, and management of incontinence. She is the author of the books, *The Urinary Incontinence Sourcebook, Managing and Treating Urinary Incontinence* (1st and 2nd editions), *Overcoming Overactive Bladder*, and a co-author of *Fast Facts: Bladder Disorders*.

Christine Norton, PhD, RN

Christine Norton is a nurse who has worked with people with incontinence for over thirty years in a variety of settings. She is Nurse Consultant, bowel control, at St. Mark's Hospital in London, which specializes in helping people with bowel (fecal) incontinence. Chris is also Professor of Clinical Nursing Innovation at Bucks New University & Imperial College

Healthcare NHS Trust, London. She has done extensive research on ways of helping people with fecal incontinence, as well as teaching nationally and internationally. Professor Norton has chaired the UK national and international guideline groups on managing fecal incontinence.

Rick Rader, MD

Dr. Rader is the Director of the Morton J. Kent Habitation Center at Orange Grove Center (Chattanooga, TN) where he is responsible for identifying innovative programs addressing the future medical problems of people aging with intellectual and developmental disabilities. He is the Editor in Chief of *Exceptional Parent Magazine* and the Vice President of Public Policy and Advocacy at the American Academy of Developmental Medicine and Dentistry, as well as a board member of the American Association on Health and Disability. Dr. Rader has published over 200 articles in the field of disabilities and health. He is cross-trained in internal medicine and medical anthropology.

Ronald H. Rozensky, PhD

Dr. Rozensky is a long-time consultant to the Simon Foundation for Continence, including working on the Foundation's initial strategic plan, its Prevention Conference, its first Stigma Conference, and on quality of life research in incontinence. He is a professor in the Department of Clinical and Health Psychology in the College of Public Health & Health Professions at the University of Florida where he also served as department chair and then Associate Dean for International Programs. He is board certified in both clinical psychology and clinical health psychology and has published five textbooks on clinical work with patients with various medical problems.

Anita Saltmarche, RN, BScN, MHSc

Ms. Saltmarche has over 25 years of experience in a variety of positions and across many different health care settings. Her clinical and research focus includes urinary incontinence, developing outpatient Geriatric Continence Clinics, and determining the position of continence nurse clinicians in long-term care. Anita developed the first Nurse Continence Advisor course in Canada. She is a founding member of the Canadian Continence Foundation (formerly Simon Canada), working first as a board member and as the elected President of the Foundation.

Steven M. Tovian, PhD

Dr. Tovian has contributed chapters in Cheryle Gartley's and the Simon Foundation's book, *Managing Incontinence: A Guide to Living with Loss of Bladder Control.* He is Associate Professor of Psychiatry and Behavioral Sciences at the Feinberg School of Medicine at Northwestern University. Currently he is in independent practice in Highland Park, Illinois. For over twenty years he served as Director of Health Psychology at the NorthShore University Health Systems Medical Group in Evanston, Illinois. He is board certified in both clinical psychology and clinical health psychology and has co-authored two textbooks and over twenty book chapters and articles on clinical work with medical patients.

Further Reading

EDITOR'S NOTE: Among the following sampling of recently published books on incontinence, we hope that you will find a title or two that will entice you to read more about the cures and treatments available for incontinence today. This list of recent publications is far from inclusive because more is being discovered and written about this topic as interest in cure and treatment expands. Nor does placement on this list mean an endorsement of either the book or the content. These books were not screened by the editors. Rather, we simply wanted to provide you a list that would highlight the breadth of the subject in order to help you get started on becoming an expert regarding misbehaving bladders and bowels and to illustrate that there is help and hope for new cures and treatments in the future. The ISBN number will help your bookstore to locate the book if you want to order it.

7 Steps to Normal Bladder Control:
Simple, Practical Tips & Techniques for Staying Dry
By Elizabeth Vierck
Publisher: Harbor Press, Inc. (1998)
ISBN-13: 978-0936197296

100 Questions and Answers about Overactive Bladder and Urinary Incontinence
By Pamela Ellsworths
Publisher: Jones and Bartlett Publishers (2005)
ISBN-13: 978-0763745462

American College of Physicians Home Medical Guide:
Urinary Incontinence in Women
By Christopher N. Martyn and C. Gale
Publisher: DK ADULT (2000)
ISBN-13: 978-0789441713

The Bathroom Key: A Treatment Plan to Put an End to Incontinence
By Kim Perelli and Kathryn Kassai
Publisher: Demos Health (2012)
ISBN-13: 978-1936303212

Beyond Kegels
By Janet A. Hulme
Publisher: Phoenix Publishing (2008)
ISBN-13: 978-1928812173

The Big Secret, Incontinence
By Sophia Kangarlu and Anita Kangarlu
Publisher: Xlibris Corp. (2010)
ISBN-13:978-1453537664

Bladder and Bowel Problems: Taking Control
By Kerry Lee
Publisher: Age Concern England (2005)
ISBN-13: 978-0862423865

Bladder Control Is No Accident: A Woman's Guide
By Dorothy B. Smith
Publisher: Deschutes Medical Products Inc (2001)
ISBN-13: 978-0970868602

Bowel Continence Nursing
By Christine Norton and Sonya Chelvanayagam
Publisher: Beaconsfield Publishers Ltd (2004)
ISBN-13: 9780906584521

Bowel Control
By Christine Norton and Michael A. Kamm
Publisher: Beaconsfield Publishers Ltd (1999)
ISBN-13: 9780906584491

British Medical Association: Incontinence in Women
By Tony Smith
Publisher: Dorling Kindersley Publishers Ltd (1999)
ISBN-13: 978-0751306729

Conquering Incontinence: A New and Physical Approach to a Freer Lifestyle
By Peter Dornan
Publisher: Allen & Unwin (2004)
ISBN-13: 978-1741141443

Conquering Bladder and Prostate Problems:
The Authoritative Guide for Men and Women
By Jerry Blaivas
Publisher: Da Capo Press (2001)
ISBN-13: 978-0738204390

Coping with Incontinence: Overcoming Common Problems
By Joan Gomez
Publisher: Sheldon Press (2004)
ISBN-13: 978-0859699006

A Crack in the Mask, The Felt Sense Method®,
A Humanistic Approach for Managing Incontinence
By Jaki Nett
Publisher: Neuter Bird Press (2010)
ISBN-13: 978-0615352206

Free Yourself from Incontinence: Your Bladder Guide
By Susan L Jackson
Publisher: Wellness Forward (2009)
ISBN-13: 978-0982268209

Harvard Medical School Better Bladder and Bowel Control
By May M. Wakamatsu, Joseph A. Grocela, and Liliana Bordeianou
Publisher: Harvard Medical School (2009)
ISBN-13: 978-1933812595

Heal Pelvic Pain: The Proven Stretching, Strengthening, and Nutrition Program for Relieving Pain, Incontinence, IBS, and Other Symptoms Without Surgery
By Amy Stein
Publisher: McGraw-Hill; 1st edition (2008)
ISBN-13: 978-0071546560

Incontinence: A Time to Heal with Yoga and Acupressure: A Six Week Exercise Program for People with Simple Stress Urinary Incontinence
By Dawn R. Mahowald and Emmey A. Ripoll
Publisher: AuthorHouse (2006)
ISBN-13: 978-1418452933

The Incontinence Solution: Answers for Women of All Ages
By William Parker, Amy Rosenman, and Rachel Parker
Publisher: Touchstone; Original Edition (2002)
ISBN-13: 978-0743215879

Keeping Control: A Practical Guide to the Prevention and Treatment of Female Incontinence
By Jane Smith, Raj Persad, Phillip Smith, and Ann Winder
Publisher: Random House UK (2001)
ISBN-13: 978-0091852191

Keeping Control: Understanding and Overcoming Fecal Incontinence (A Johns Hopkins Press Health Book)
By Marvin M. Schuster and Jacqueline Wehmueller
Publisher: The Johns Hopkins University Press (1994)
ISBN-13: 978-0801849169

Managing and Treating Urinary Incontinence
By Diane Kaschak Newman
Publisher: Health Professions Press (2008)
ISBN-13: 978-1932529210

Mayo Clinic on Managing Incontinence: Practical Strategies for Improving Bladder and Bowel Control
Paul Pettit (Editor)
Publisher: Mayo Clinic (2005)
ASIN: B000ZST3SW

Natural Treatments for Urinary Incontinence
By Rita Elkins
Publisher: Woodland Publishing; Booklet Edition (2000)
ISBN-13: 978-1580540858

Overcoming Incontinence: A Straightforward Guide to Your Options
By Mary Dierich and Felecia Froe
Publisher: Wiley; 1st edition (2000)
ISBN-13: 978-0471347958

Overcoming Urinary Incontinence: A Woman's Guide to Treatment
By Michael H. Safir, Clay N. Boyd, and Tony E. Pinson
Publisher: Addicus Books (2008)
ISBN-13: 978-1886039872

Prostate Cancer Survivors Speak Their Minds: Advice on Options, Treatments, and Aftereffects
By Arthur L. Burnett and Norman Morris
Publisher: Wiley (2010)
ISBN-13: 978-0470578810

Questions & Answers About Overactive Bladder
By Pamela Ellsworth and Alan Wein
Publisher: Jones & Bartlett Publishers (2009)
ISBN-13: 978-0763771980

Regaining Bladder Control: What Every Woman Needs to Know
By Rebecca G. Rogers, Janet Yagoda Shagam, and Shelley Kleinschmidt
Publisher: Prometheus Books (2006)
ISBN-13: 978-1591024163

Saving the Whole Woman: Natural Alternatives to Surgery for Pelvic Organ Prolapse and Urinary Incontinence
By Christine Ann Kent
Publisher: Bridgeworks, Inc. (2008)
ISBN-13: 978-0970144010

A Seat on the Aisle, Please! The Essential Guide to Urinary Tract Problems in Women
By Elizabeth Kavaler
Publisher: Springer (2006)
ISBN-10: 0387955097

Urinary Incontinence: A Practical Guide for People with Bladder Control Problems, Their Careers and Health Care Professionals
By David Fonda
Publisher: Ausmed Publications (2004)
ISBN-13: 978-0868398082

A Woman's Guide to Regaining Bladder Control:
Everything You Need to Know for the Diagnosis and Cure of Incontinence
By Eric S. Rovener, Alan J. Wein, and Donna Caruso
Publisher: M. Evans & Company (2004)
ISBN-13: 978-1590770405

A Woman's Guide to Urinary Incontinence: A Johns Hopkins Press Health Book
By Rene Genadry
Publisher: The Johns Hopkins University Press (2007)
ISBN-13: 978-0801887338

Women's Waterworks: Curing Incontinence
By Pauline E. Chiarelli
Publisher: Khera Publications, Limited (2004)
ISBN-10: 0964071908

You Go Girl...But Only When You Want To!
By Missy D. Lavender and Dorothy B. Smith
Publisher: Women's Health Foundation (2007)
ISBN-13: 978-0979687600

Glossary

Anal canal: Passageway between the rectum and the outside of the body.

Anal plug: A small foam plug inserted into the anus to control stool leakage.

Anal sphincter: The rings of muscle around the anus that keep the sphincter closed and help to maintain bowel control.

Anorectal physiological studies: Specialized tests of the nerves and muscles of the rectum and anus.

Anus: The opening at the lower end of the rectum, through which stool is passed.

Bedside commode: A portable toilet used by individuals who have difficulty getting to standard facilities.

Behavioral techniques: Specific interventions designed to alter the relationship between the person's symptoms and behavior and/or environment for the treatment of bladder or bowel problems.

Benign prostatic hyperplasia (BPH): A common disorder in men over the age of fifty that is characterized by enlargement of the prostate gland, which may press against the urethra and interfere with the flow of urine.

Biofeedback therapy: A behavioral technique in which a person learns how to consciously control involuntary responses such as muscle contractions. The person receives a visual, auditory, or tactile signal (the feedback) that indicates how well the person's muscles are responding to the commands of the person's nervous system.

Bladder: A muscular organ that lies in the pelvis and is supported by the pelvic floor muscles. The bladder is often referred to as the "detrusor muscle," which is the smooth muscle layer of the bladder.

Bladder control: Ability to control urination.

Bladder diary or record: A daily record of bladder habits, voiding, episodes of incontinence, fluid intake, etc.

Bladder or bowel training: A behavioral technique that educates the person on strategies to resist or inhibit the sensation of urgency, to postpone voiding or defecating.

Cesarean section (C-section): Operation for birth of a baby through an abdominal incision.

Call to stool: The feeling that the bowel needs emptying.

Catheter: A narrow, flexible tube that can be inserted through the urethra into the bladder.

Catheterization: A procedure in which a catheter is passed through the urethra and into the bladder for the purpose of draining urine and performing diagnostic tests of bladder or urethral function.

Clean intermittent catheterization: Insertion of a clean catheter into the bladder at regular intervals.

Codeine phosphate: Medicine to treat diarrhea or loose stools.

Collection bag: Leg bag or bedside collector, designed to collect urine by gravity, which is connected by tubing to an indwelling or external catheter.

Colon: The large intestines or large bowel which absorbs water from the waste from food that your body cannot use, and forms it into stools.

Colonoscopy: Examination of the colon using a tiny camera on the end of a flexible tube, which allows the doctor to inspect the wall of the bowel from the inside.

Colostomy: A surgically created opening of the bowel on the abdominal wall.

Condom (external) catheters: A condom-like device placed over the penis to allow bladder drainage and collection of urine. Devices are made from latex rubber, polyvinyl, or silicone, are secured on the shaft of the penis by some form of adhesive, and are connected to urine collecting bags by a tube.

Constipation: The experience of infrequent or hard stools that are difficult or uncomfortable to pass.

Continence: The ability to exercise voluntary control over urination or defecation.

Crohn or Crohn's disease: A disease of the bowel in which patches of the bowel wall become inflamed from time to time. This can lead to pain, diarrhea, and sometimes passing blood. In most cases it can be controlled by modern medicines.

Cystitis: Irritation or inflammation (swelling) of the bladder usually caused by an infection.

Defecation: Passing a stool or having a bowel movement (BM).

Detrusor: In the urinary system, the detrusor muscle is the smooth (involuntary) muscle in the wall of the bladder that contracts the bladder and expels the urine.

Diastasis: The division of the abdominal muscles from top to bottom.

Dysuria: Painful or difficult urination, most frequently caused by infection or inflammation.

Electrical stimulation: The use of electric current to stimulate or inhibit the pelvic floor muscles or their nerve supply in order to reduce bladder or bowel symptoms; often referred to as E-Stim.

Enema: Liquid inserted into the rectum through the anus to stimulate bowel emptying.

Enuresis: The uncontrolled or involuntary discharge of urine while sleeping, also called bed-wetting.

Estrogen: A hormone produced primarily by the ovaries. Estrogen is believed to play a major role in maintaining the strength and tone of the muscles of the pelvic floor.

Evacuation: Another word for bowel movement.

External anal sphincter: The voluntary muscle around the anus that you can squeeze to delay passing stool.

External urethral sphincter: A voluntary muscle surrounding the urethra that opens and closes to hold urine in or let it drain out of the bladder.

Feces: Bowel motions, the waste products of the digestive system, also known as "stool."

Fiber: The indigestible part of plants (fruit and vegetables) in the food we eat, which forms a large part of the feces. Fiber helps to hold water in the feces, making them softer and easier to pass.

Fissure: A small split in the lining of the anal canal, which can be very painful, particularly when opening the bowels.

Flatus: Gas or wind produced in the bowel, mostly as a result of the normal activity of bacteria in the bowel.

Foley catheter: A catheter that is inserted into the bladder through the urethra for continuous emptying of the bladder; also called an indwelling catheter.

Functional incontinence: This is urinary or fecal leakage that occurs when the urinary or fecal body systems, respectively, are physiologically working fine. The incontinence is, instead, the result of mobility challenges in getting to a bathroom and/or removing clothing in a reasonable amount of time.

Gastro-colic reflex: Automatic increase in bowel contractions in response to eating or drinking. This can lead to a mass movement of stool in the colon, and a call to stool shortly afterwards.

Habit training: A behavioral technique that uses scheduled toileting at regular intervals on a planned basis to prevent incontinence.

Hematuria: The presence of blood in urine.

Hemorrhoids: Enlargement of the normal cushions of blood vessels inside the anus. These may bleed and cause pain when opening the bowels.

Hemorrhoidectomy: Surgical removal of troublesome hemorrhoids.

Hesitancy: Difficulty in starting the urine stream.

Hirschsprung's disease: Rare disease that is congenital (you are born with it). The nerves at the lower end of the rectum fail to develop, leading to severe constipation.

Ileostomy: A surgically created opening of the small bowel onto the wall of the abdomen.

Imodium: Medicine to treat diarrhea or loose stool; also called loperamide.

Impaction: Bowel is overloaded with stool, causing a blockage This blockage may cause irritation of the bowel wall and mucus and loose stool may leak around the blockage and be mistaken for diarrhea.

Incontinence: Loss of control of the contents of the bowel (fecal or bowel incontinence) or of the bladder (urinary incontinence). A person may have urinary or fecal incontinence or both (sometimes called double incontinence.)

Indwelling catheters: Catheters that are inserted into the bladder to drain urine; may also be referred to as a Foley catheter.

Inflammatory Bowel Disease (IBD): Common name for ulcerative colitis and Crohn's disease.

Intermittency: Interruption of urinary stream while voiding (stops and starts).

Intermittent catheterization: The use of catheters inserted through the urethra into the bladder at regular intervals throughout the day to drain the bladder.

Internal anal sphincter: Inner ring of muscle around the anal canal. This muscle works automatically to keep the anus closed at all times except when you need to pass a stool.

Intractable: Not resolving or resistant to treatment.

Irritable Bowel Syndrome (IBS): Bowel disorder that causes an irregular and unpredictable bowel habit, often constipation alternating with loose stools, and usually with abdominal discomfort or pain.

Kidney: One of two paired organs (the kidneys) that continually filter the blood to separate out waste products, which are combined with excess water to form urine.

Kidney infection: A urinary tract infection that includes the kidneys, and is also known as pyelonephritis.

Laxative: Medicine to treat constipation.

Leg bag: A bag that attaches to the leg with straps to collect urine from an indwelling catheter (male or female) or from a male external catheter (or condom catheter).

Lomotil: Medicine to treat diarrhea or loose stools.

Loperamide: Medicine to treat diarrhea or loose stools.

Manometry: Tests to measure pressures in the muscles of the rectum and anus.

Mass movements: Waves of activity in the colon propelling stool large distances toward the anus.

Meatus: The opening to the urethra.

Micturition: The act of voiding urine; urination.

Mixed urinary incontinence: The combination of urge and stress urinary incontinence.

Nervous system: The voluntary and involuntary nervous system are composed of the brain, the spinal cord, and the sensory nerves, which provide messages to the brain from the body, and motor nerves, which provide messages from the brain to the muscles and which help muscles function.

Neurogenic bladder: A bladder that is overactive or underactive as the result of a neurological condition, such as diabetes, stroke, or spinal cord injury.

Nocturia: Being awakened at night by the urge to urinate.

Nocturnal enuresis: Involuntary nocturnal urination during sleep.

Overactive bladder: A condition characterized by involuntary bladder contractions during the bladder filling phase, causing incontinence or a frequent urge to urinate.

Overflow incontinence: The involuntary loss of urine associated with over-distension of the bladder. This may result from urinary retention caused by obstruction of the urethra.

Passive soiling: Losing stool through the anus without feeling the urge to open the bowels.

Pelvic floor muscles: The hammock of muscles that support the bladder, bowel, and in women the vagina. These muscles assist in maintaining continence by supporting the pelvic organs.

Pelvic muscle exercises: A behavioral technique that requires repetitive active exercise of the pubococcygeus muscle to improve urinary or bowel control by strengthening the pelvic muscles. These are also called Kegel exercises or pelvic floor exercises.

Pelvis: Ring of bones at the lower end of the (body's) trunk which encircles the pelvic organs.

Penile clamp: Device used to put direct pressure on the urethra causing it to remain closed until the device is removed and the bladder is allowed to drain.

Perineum: Area between the anus and vagina in women, and anus and base of the penis in men.

Pessary: An appliance like a diaphragm, which is available in many sizes and is placed in the vagina to hold a prolapsed, or dropped, organ in place.

Polyuria: Producing an excessive amount of urine. It can be a result of uncontrolled diabetes mellitus or from the administration of a diuretic.

Post-anal repair: Surgical repair of the muscles behind the anus.

Post-void residual (PVR) volume: The amount of fluid remaining in the bladder immediately after voiding.

Posterior tibial nerve stimulation (PTNS): A technique of electrical neuromodulation for the treatment of bladder or bowel dysfunction in patients who have failed behavioral and/or pharmacologic therapies.

Prolapse: The dropping of the pelvic organs (e.g., uterus, rectum, urethra, and/or bladder) into the vagina; also referred to as POP (Pelvic Organ Prolapse). *See* also rectal prolapse.

Prostate: A circular-shaped gland found only in men that surrounds the urethra between the bladder and the pelvic floor.

Pruritus ani: Severe itching and irritation of the skin around the anus.

Rectal prolapse: Laxity of the wall of muscle of the rectum so that it comes down through the anus.

Rectum: The lowest part of the bowel where stools are held until the toilet is reached.

Retention: Inability to empty urine from the bladder, which can be caused by a bladder that does not contract or obstruction of the urethra.

Risk factor: Condition that makes a person more susceptible to a specific disease.

Scheduled toileting: Assistance to toilet or use of bedpan or urinal offered on a fixed schedule, for example, every two to four hours.

Self-catheterization: The process of emptying the bladder with an intermittent catheter.

Small bowel: The small intestines, which run from the stomach down to the colon and are responsible for digesting the food and absorbing the nutrients from it into the bloodstream.

Stool: Bowel motions, the waste products of the digestive system, also known as feces.

Stress urinary incontinence: A form of urinary incontinence characterized by the involuntary loss of urine from the urethra during physical exertion; for example, during coughing, exercising, laughing, etc.

Stricture: The narrowing of a passage within the body. A urethral stricture is the narrowing of the urethra.

Suppositories: Small cone inserted through the anus into the rectum to lubricate or stimulate bowel emptying.

Suprapubic: Above the pubic bone.

Suprapubic catheter: A catheter that is inserted through the skin above the pubic bone and into the bladder for drainage of urine.

Timed voiding: Planned trips to the bathroom to urinate.

Ulcerative colitis: An inflammatory disease of the colon that can cause diarrhea and abdominal pain.

Ultrasound: Use of sound waves to create images of the internal organs of the body.

Underactive bladder: A bladder with an overly large capacity that overfills with urine. Loss of sensation due to this filling action results in a bladder that does not contract forcefully enough, and small amounts of urine dribble from the urethra.

Ureters: Two very thin muscular tubes that carry urine from the kidneys to the bladder.

Urethra: Narrow tube through which urine flows from the bladder to the outside of the body.

Urethral obstruction: Blockage of the urethra causing difficulty with urination; usually caused by a stricture or by an enlarged prostate gland in men.

Urge: Sensation from the bladder producing the normal desire to void.

Urge incontinence: Involuntary and accidental loss of urine when the person is aware of the need to get to the bathroom, but is not able to hold on long enough to get there. Usually it is associated with an abrupt and strong desire to void (urgency).

Urgency: A strong, intense, and often sudden desire to void.

Urinalysis: A diagnostic test to examine the contents of urine to determine the presence of infection, to diagnose metabolic disease, and/or to obtain information about kidney function.

Urinary incontinence (UI): Involuntary or accidental loss of urine sufficient to be a problem.

Urinary tract infection (UTI): An infection in the urinary tract caused by bacteria. Infection of the bladder, better known as cystitis, is more common in women, mainly because of the much shorter urethra. In men, infection is usually associated with obstruction to the flow of urine, such as prostate gland enlargement.

Urinate (urinating): To void or to pass urine.

Urination: The act of passing urine.

Urine: A mixture of waste products and water produced by the kidneys.

Urodynamic tests: Tests that measurement the function of the bladder.

Vagina: Also known as the birth canal. The vagina is a collapsible tube of smooth muscle with its opening located between the urethral orifice and the anal sphincter of women.

Voiding: Another word for urinating, sometimes called "peeing" or "passing water."

The Simon Foundation
for Continence

Managing Life with Incontinence is brought to you by the Simon Foundation for Continence, a U.S.-based nonprofit organization. It was founded in 1982 and incorporated in 1983 during the "dark ages" of incontinence, a period when the stigma surrounding incontinence made the symptom of incontinence so taboo that there were: no overhead signs in retail aisles announcing incontinence products; no books on the subject in libraries; no television or radio commercials advertising medications or absorbent products; a complete absence of articles in major magazines or newspapers; and little, if anything, taught about incontinence in medical and nursing schools.

In the midst of this information void and complete lack of help, the Simon Foundation began its mission to bring the topic of incontinence into the open, remove the stigma surrounding incontinence, and provide help and hope to individuals with incontinence, their families, and the professionals who provide their care.

In 1985 the Simon Foundation produced *Managing Incontinence: A Guide to Living with Loss of Bladder Control*, the first book written for the general public on the topic of incontinence which was translated into Spanish, Japanese, and British English. This book was the groundwork for an extensive worldwide media tour resulting in groundbreaking articles in magazines such as *TIME Magazine* and appearances on popular television shows such as Good Morning Australia. Since then, the Simon Foundation has been one of the United States' foremost advocacy organizations representing people with incontinence.

As the news of Simon's work expanded beyond America's borders we: co-founded Simon Canada (now The Canadian Continence Foundation); addressed members of the Australian government in Canberra; met with a team from the Japanese Ministry of Health in Tokyo; and co-founded the Continence Promotion Committee of the International Continence Society.

Other groundbreaking endeavors have included conferences that are developed by the Simon Foundation on topics not typically covered at incontinence related medical and nursing meetings. This is done to shine a spotlight on areas of great importance to individuals with incontinence. For example, the Foundation organized Prevention 97, the first conference to focus upon the prevention of incontinence. Held in London, England in 1997, this meeting brought together experts from New Zealand, Norway, England, Australia, Canada, the Netherlands, Denmark, Singapore, Austria, Japan, and the United States to highlight what was known about prevention and create a call to action for further research in this then neglected area. Other Simon initiated groundbreaking conferences include: Defeating Stigma in Healthcare (2003) and Innovating for Continence: The Engineering Challenge (2007, 2009, 2011), which is a unique biennial meeting that brings together a widely diverse group of stakeholders whose goal is to increase the rate of innovation for new products and devices for the management of incontinence.

The Foundation was named after the grandfather of its founder, Cheryle Gartley. Simon escaped under gunfire from the communism he despised to the freedom of America that he adored. He spoke seven languages fluently and yet seemed to know only one response to every complaint his teenage granddaughter could express, and the response always began with, "But young lady, in this country everything can be changed." The Simon Foundation was named in honor of that belief.

Most people working in nonprofits, no matter what their cause, but certainly those of us addressing devastating health conditions, always hope to create sufficient change to work ourselves out of a job. It is no different here at the Simon Foundation. However, until that day arrives, the Foundation continues to help individuals overcome the impact of their incontinence and live the life of their choice.

In the 27 years since the Foundation's first book was published, a lot has changed in the world: there is much easier access to information through the Internet, and there are far more treatment and management options available than ever before. But one thing has not changed: people are still living with incontinence and the fear, shame, and embarrassment that accompany it.

In this new book, the Simon Foundation for Continence hopes that you'll find the support that you need to "manage life with incontinence."

Index

A

Absorbent products, 159-162
Adaptive devices, 162-163, 182
Aging
  effects on incontinence, 34, 194-195
Alcohol, 41, 193
Anal incontinence, *See* Fecal incontinence
Anal plugs, 161-162
Anal sphincters, 58
Antidiarrhea drugs, 64
Anxiety
  in incontinence, 77-78
  reducing, 78, 81-82
    thought stopping technique, 78
Appointments with health care professionals,
  108-116
Artificial sphincters, 46, 65
Assertiveness training, 80-81

B

Barrier creams and wipes, 165, 184
Bedwetting, *See* Nocturnal enuresis
Behavioral interventions
  in constipation and fecal incontinence, 43
  in nocturnal enuresis, 42-43
  in urinary incontinence, 40-42, 44-45
Benign prostatic hyperplasia (BPH), 31, 36, 193
Biofeedback, 63, 192
Bladder
  capacity, 33-34
    aging effects, 34
  emptying, 33-34
  function, normal, 29-34
  innervation, 32-33
  urge to void, 33-34
  See also Voiding
Bladder diaries, 38-39, 109-110
Bladder re-education (retraining), 44-45
Bladder training, 3, 5
Body image, 71-73, 82-83
  managing, 77-83
    assertiveness training, 80-81
    progressive muscle relaxation, 81
    self-talk, 78-80
Body image, altered, 72-83
  in incontinence, 72-73
  personal response, 73
  sexual response, 74
  social response, 74-75, 122-123
Bowel control, 55-59

Bowel Control *(continued)*
  See also Defecation; Fecal incontinence
Bowel habits
  normal, 43, 57-59
Bowel incontinence, *See* Fecal incontinence
Bowel irrigation, 64
Bowel movement, *See* Defecation
Bowel training (retraining), 60-61
BPH, *See* Benign prostatic hyperplasia

C

Caffeine, 41, 65, 193
Carbonated drinks, 41
Cleansing, 163, 184
Clothing, 180, 182, 184-185
Colon, 56
Communicating
  at work, 96
  concern level, 113-114
  conversation goal setting, 93, 139
  impact of incontinence on life style, 110-111
  in embarrassing situations, 96-98
  in personal situations, 98
  symptoms of incontinence, 111-113
  terminology, 93-95, 138-139
  tracking conversation habits, 150
  with people you know, 91-98
  with use of questions, 114-115
  with your health care professional, 105-116
Condom catheters, 160
Constipation
  causes, 59-60
Continence organizations, 199-209
Coping strategies, 75-77, 82-83, 124
  guidelines, 77
Creative problem solving, 176-178
  brainstorming, 176-177
  problem elements, 174

D

Defecation
  at convenient time, 64
  awareness of need, 57-59
  controlled, 63-64
  digital assistance, 64
  ignoring urge, 58-59
    constipation, 59
  manners and customs, 2-3
  normal, 58-59

Questionnaire

Please help us to better understand the needs of individuals with incontinence by filling out the following questionnaire and returning it to **The Simon Foundation, Post Office Box 815, Wilmette, Illinois 60091, USA.** Alternatively if you prefer to give us your input on line, you will find this questionnaire at **www.simonfoundation.org.**

ABOUT YOU:

Age: ____ Sex: ____

I have had incontinence for ____years.

I have: ___urinary incontinence ___bowel incontinence ___both

My urinary incontinence is: ___stress ___urgency ___mixed ___overactive bladder

___overflow ___functional

The reason for my incontinence is _____

_____

I ___have ___have not consulted a doctor about my incontinence.

If you have consulted a physician how soon after this symptom began did you schedule an appointment? _____

If you have not yet sought help, please share the reason why you haven't.

_____

_____

ABOUT INCONTINENCE AND ITS IMPACT:

On a scale of 1 -10 (10 being the most impact) how would you rate the impact of your incontinence on your quality of life? _____

What are the top three changes that you have made in your life because of incontinence?

1. _____

2. _____

3. _____

continued on next page

Questionnaire, *continued*

What needs do you have concerning incontinence which are not currently being met?

_____

_____

ABOUT THIS BOOK:

I purchased this book:

_____ directly from The Simon Foundation

_____ from an online book retailer

_____ at a bookstore

_____ it was a gift

What did you find the most helpful in this book? _____

What was the least helpful? _____

On a scale of 1-10 (10 being the highest) please rate this book? _____

If you would like news from The Simon Foundation for Continence, or are willing to participate in future surveys, please provide your contact details:

_____ I would prefer to be contacted by mail:

   Name: _____

   Street Address: _____

   City, State, Zip Code: _____

   Country: _____

_____ I would prefer to be contacted by email at:

_____